Children's High Dependency Nursing

Children's High Dependency Nursing

Edited by

Andrea Cockett
RGN, RSCN, ENB 160 998,
BSc (Hons) Child Health, PGCEA
Independent Paediatric Nurse Consultant

and

Helen Day
RGN, RSCN, ENB 415, DipN, BSc (Hons) Child Health,
MSc Nursing (Paediatric Advanced Nurse Practitioner)
Head of Care, InVent Health Ltd

WILEY-BLACKWELL

A John Wiley & Sons, Ltd., Publication

This edition first published 2010
© 2010 John Wiley & Sons, Ltd

Wiley-Blackwell is an imprint of John Wiley & Sons, formed by the merger of Wiley's global
Scientific, Technical and Medical business with Blackwell Publishing.

Registered office
John Wiley & Sons Ltd, The Atrium, Southern Gate, Chichester, West Sussex, PO19 8SQ,
United Kingdom

Editorial office
John Wiley & Sons Ltd, The Atrium, Southern Gate, Chichester, West Sussex, PO19 8SQ,
United Kingdom

For details of our global editorial offices, for customer services and for information about
how to apply for permission to reuse the copyright material in this book please see our
website at www.wiley.com/wiley-blackwell.

The right of the author to be identified as the author of this work has been asserted in
accordance with the Copyright, Designs and Patents Act 1988.

Library of Congress Cataloging-in-Publication Data

Children's high dependency nursing / edited by Andrea Cockett and Helen Day.
    p. ; cm.
  Includes bibliographical references.
  ISBN 978-0-470-51716-1 (cloth)
  1. Pediatric nursing. 2. Pediatric intensive care. 3. Intensive care nursing.
I. Cockett, Andrea. II. Day, Helen, RGN.
  [DNLM: 1. Pediatric Nursing–methods. 2. Subacute Care–methods. WY 159 C5372
2010]
  RJ245.C4775 2010
  618.92'0028–dc22

               2009023913

A catalogue record for this book is available from the British Library.

Set in 10 on 12 pt Palatino by SNP Best-set Typesetter Ltd., Hong Kong
Printed and bound in Singapore by Fabulous Printers Pte Ltd

1 2010

Contents

Contributors

Leanne Burns
BSc (Hons) Children's Nursing; Senior Sister, Thomas Cook Children's Intensive Care, King's College Hospital
Leanne qualified as a paediatric nurse from Leeds University and has worked for several years within paediatric intensive care at King's College Hospital. Following completion of a postgraduate intensive care course, she developed an interest in advanced nursing practice and is due to complete an MSc in this field. Recently Leanne has moved out of the intensive care environment and she now jointly manages a specialist paediatric liver and gastrointestinal ward. Leanne has contributed to several other publications within paediatric nursing.

Sheena Carson
RGN, RN Child, BSc Children's Nursing, Masters in Academic Practice
Sheena has been working as a Lecturer in Child Health at King's College London for the past four years, with the majority of her teaching focusing on the emergency care of critically ill children and young people for both undergraduate and post-qualification students. Prior to this, she spent eight years working in the specialist area of paediatric accident & emergency nursing within two central London departments.

Louise Clark
BA, MSc, SRN, RN(LD), PGCAP
Louise Clark is a Lecturer in Intellectual Impairment and Mental Health at the Florence Nightingale School of Nursing & Midwifery, King's College London. She is responsible for the coordination of education in intellectual impairment throughout the school, at undergraduate and postgraduate levels, and has published widely in her specialist area.

Andrea Cockett
RGN, RSCN, ENB 160 998, BSc (Hons) Child Health, PGCEA; Independent Paediatric Nurse Consultant
Andrea has spent the majority of her career working with children with cardiac disease or in intensive care environments. For the last nine years she was a Lecturer in Child Health at King's College London, holding the post of joint Head of Department. She left this post in 2007 to spend more time with her family and currently undertakes both voluntary and paid work in the field of child health.

Helen Day
RGN, RSCN, ENB 415, DipN, BSc (Hons) Child Health, MSc Nursing (Paediatric Advanced Nurse Practitioner); Head of Care, InVent Health Ltd
Helen's career has been varied and she has worked in primary and secondary care settings for the NHS, independent and third sector. After working mainly in a management and educational capacity in paediatric critical care, she is now a Consultant Nurse for InVent Health Ltd, specializing in adults and children with complex needs. Her achievements include the development of one of the first paediatric critical care outreach services and writing and presenting widely on the nature of nursing and advancing nursing practice in critical care.

Paula Kelly
PhD, PGCE, RNT, MSc, RSCN, RGN, BA (Hons); Nurse Consultant, Community Children's Nursing Service, NHS Newham Community Health and Care Services
Paula is an experienced children's nurse and the focus of her clinical work has been caring for children in the home setting. This has included leading generalist community children's nursing services, and specialist work in oncology and HIV. This clinical work led to a concern to identify, through research, the impact of these experiences on family life for children with long-term and life-limiting health difficulties. Her doctoral study focused on the impact of children's cancer on experiences of childhood and parenthood in a minority ethnic context. After a considerable period in academic nursing and as a nurse advisor to the Health Ombudsman, Paula is now linking clinical work with research and service development in a newly established Nurse Consultant role.

Deborah Lynn

BA (Hons) Child Branch; Senior Sister, Diana Team, Complex Care and Palliative Care, Community Children's Nursing Service; NHS Newham, Community Health and Care Services

Deborah Lynn is an experienced paediatric nurse, who has worked in both hospital and community settings. Her focus in the acute setting has been paediatric oncology including palliative care, while in the community she has focused on specialist work in epilepsy, as well as generic children's community nursing. She is currently the lead for the palliative care/complex care service in Newham PCT, in which the majority of clients are children with high dependency needs. Her degree dissertation study explored the child's concept of death, through which she developed her interest in paediatric palliative care.

Lynne Wainwright

RGN, RSCN, NNEB, DipHE (Neonatal Nursing), ENB 998, ENB 405, Enhanced Neonatal Nursing Practice, MSc

Lynne trained at Charles West School of Nursing, Great Ormond Street Hospital, and the Hammersmith Hospital and was a Staff Nurse on the Private Patient Unit for ten years before moving to the Neonatal Intensive Care Unit at Great Ormond Street Hospital. She has worked on the Neonatal Intensive Care Unit at University Hospital Lewisham for ten years, the last seven as Practice Development Nurse. During that time she also had a three-year part-time secondment to King's College London as Clinical Skills Facilitator for Child Branch Nursing. Lynne's particular interests are neonatal nutrition and ventilation.

Joan Walters

BSc (Hons) Health Studies, MSc Social Anthropology of Nursing, Registered Nurse (Adult), Registered Nurse (Child), Fellow of the Higher Education Academy, ENB N08 Haemoglobinopathy Nursing, ENB 240 Paediatric Oncology Nursing, ENB 870 Research Awareness, ENB 998 Teaching & Assessing, Certificate in Coaching (Caledonian University); Senior Practitioner Lecturer, Child Health, Variety Club Children's Hospital, King's College Hospital NHS Foundation Trust and Florence Nightingale School of Nursing & Midwifery, King's College, London

Joan trained as a children's nurse at King's College Hospital and developed an interest in haematology and oncology after working in and then managing the specialist ward. Within the Trust, Joan is part of the Senior Nurse Management Team and the Lead Nurse for the Child Health Practice Development Team. At the college, Joan leads on the Child Branch course 'Children and young people with chronic illness.'

She also leads the post-qualification course on haemoglobinopathy nursing. Joan has been one of the national trainers for the NHS Haemoglobinopathy trainers and is co-author of a parents' handbook published by the Department of Health.

Joyce Wood
RGN, RSCN, NNEB, ENB 998, ENB 405, ENB R23
Joyce trained at Liverpool John Moore University, Alder Hey Children's Hospital and Broadgreen District General Hospital. She was a Staff Nurse on the paediatric ward at the Royal Brompton Hospital for 18 months and has worked at University Hospital Lewisham as a Staff Nurse on the Neonatal Intensive Care Unit for 15 years. She also shared the post of Practice Development Nurse for 18 months.

What is high dependency care?

Helen Day and Andrea Cockett

Learning outcomes

- To develop an understanding of the definition of high dependency care and the various clinical criteria within that definition
- To develop an understanding of the potential issues and obstacles that can occur in the delivery of high dependency care
- To develop an understanding of tools to assist in the delivery of high dependency care such as early warning scores and critical care outreach

Introduction

Children's healthcare needs have changed dramatically over the last decade. The *National Service Framework for Children, Young People and Maternity Services* requires that all hospitals that admit children as inpatients must be able to provide high dependency care (Department of Health 2004a). This presents a challenge to both nursing and medical staff, particularly in NHS Trusts where high dependency and paediatric intensive care services have not been provided before. High dependency care is difficult to define and this leads to problems identifying correct nurse-to-patient ratios, nurse allocation, nursing and medical education, clinical expertise and environmental factors such as space and equipment. The Department of Health defines high dependency care as:

care provided to a child who may require closer observation and monitoring than is usually available on ordinary children's wards. High dependency is largely defined by the nature of the condition or care received and is dependent on disease, intervention or condition. (Department of Health 2002)

Little has been written about high dependency care in paediatrics; however, there has been recognition in the literature and a longstanding awareness among healthcare professionals that critically ill adult patients are to be found outside of the intensive care unit and that the care of these patients is often suboptimal (McQuillan *et al.* 1998; Goldhill *et al.* 1999a, 1999b; McGloin *et al.* 1999). More recent work revealed similar findings in paediatrics (Day *et al.* 2005; Tume 2007).

This chapter examines the background and current issues in paediatric high dependency services and presents useful findings and suggestions for future provision of paediatric high dependency care including critical care outreach and early warning systems.

What is high dependency care?

The current definition – 'care provided to a child who may require closer observation and monitoring than is usually available on ordinary children's wards' (Department of Health 1997: 7) – has led to confusion and time-consuming audits regarding what conditions and interventions should be classified as high dependency. Effective classification is necessary as it will enable appropriate care delivery by the appropriate person in the appropriate place and optimize budget and resource management. However, we do not necessarily have to redefine high dependency care as this definition encompasses clinically what may be a wide range of conditions. Two approaches may be utilized to identify high dependency patients in the clinical arena.

One approach subdivides the level 1 definition utilized by the Department of Health (Table 1.1), and the second approach, developed at King's College Hospital (Table 1.2), utilizes specific criteria and procedures to identify which children may require high dependency care and has also identified specific high-risk procedures. These criteria can be used in partnership with the high dependency classifications to organize care in other clinical settings (Tables 1.3, 1.4 and 1.5).

Table 1.1 Identifying high dependency patients – approach 1.

Identified patient level	Assessment criteria	Intervention
Level 1a	Patients who trigger a validated Early Warning Score (EWS) and whose clinical condition is deteriorating or showing no sign of improvement, and staff express concern about their clinical status	These patients may require admission to HDU based on assessment by paediatric critical care outreach nurse and local admission guidelines or continued care on ward with paediatric critical care outreach (PCCO) support if in a lead centre. Retrieval should be considered and transfer if in a district general hospital. Regional guidelines should be developed. Nurse to patient ratio 1 : 1
Level 1b	Patients who trigger EWS but their clinical condition demonstrates a trend of improvement.	These patients will probably not require admission to high dependency unit but remain on a ward with PCCO or agreed regular medical assessment and support. Nurse to patient ratio 1 : 2
Level 1c	Patients who require more frequent observations than every 60 mins, mainly those who have undergone an elective procedure which has an associated risk, e.g. liver biopsy, or those that have undergone major surgery but are clinically stable and not triggering the EWS	These patients do not require high dependency unit admission or PCCO unless, like any patient, they trigger the EWS. Nurse to patient ratio 1 : 2
Level 1d	Long-term ventilated	Should be cared for where appropriate depending on local facilities and in accordance with guidelines
Level 1e	Patients who require frequent nursing interventions, for example meeting at least two of the following criteria: >2° turns, incontinent, >2° enteral feeds or medications, agitated or disorientated and endangering themselves physically	Nurse to patient ratio 1 : 2 but will be patient specific and may require audit to facilitate effective manpower allocation

Table 1.2 King's College Hospital Referral and Transfer Guidelines for the Paediatric High-Dependency and Intensive Care Unit. Reproduced by kind permission of King's College Hospital NHS Foundation Trust.

	Paediatric High-Dependency Care Unit	**Paediatric Intensive Care Unit**
A	Upper airway obstruction with persistent symptoms/signs – requiring close observation	Upper airway obstruction – after ≥2 doses of nebulized adrenaline, or possibility of progressive deterioration/potential to total obstruction
B	Recurrent apnoeas (≥20 s each on >1 occasion)	Recurrent apnoeas with possibility of progressive deterioration
2	Acute supplemental FiO_2 requirement ≥0.5 via headbox or face mask to maintain $SaO_2 > 92\%$	Any airway intervention, or needing advanced respiratory support *other than during recovery from anaesthetic*
3	Progressive moderately severe airway or pulmonary disease with obstruction potential or risk of progression to respiratory failure	Rapidly progressive severe airway or pulmonary disease with risk of progression to total obstruction and/or respiratory failure
4	Acute severe asthma on IV bronchodilator infusion	Acute severe asthma failing to respond to therapy
C	IV fluid resuscitation >20 ml/kg and <40 ml/kg	Uncontrolled shock needing ≥40 ml/kg volume resuscitation or repeated volume or inotropes
2	Circulatory instability due to hypovolaemia	Continuous invasive cardiovascular monitoring – CV or arterial pressure
3	Non-ventilated patient requiring a stable low-dose IV inotropic or vasodilator infusion	Need for IV vasoactive drug infusions to support cardiac output or control blood pressure
4	Acute non-life-threatening dysrhythmia, or acute cardiac arrhythmia which has responded to first-line therapy (other than cardioversion)	Life-threatening dysrhythmia, or arrhythmia which fails to respond to first-line therapy, or patient requiring cardioversion or cardiac pacing
D	Acute deterioration on Glasgow Coma Scale to 9–12 requiring neurological assessment and without airway or respiratory compromise	Acute CNS depression/deterioration sufficient to compromise the airway protective reflexes/respiratory drive or high risk of progression or GCS ≤8
2	Seizures responsive to therapy with potential for respiratory compromise	Unresponsive seizures on continuous IV anticonvulsant infusion
3	Acute CNS infection or inflammation – 1ˢᵗ 12–48 hours	Acute CNS infection/inflammation with CNS/cardiorespiratory compromise
E	Nasal/face mask CPAP & $FiO_2 < 0.6$ for bronchiolitis, sickle cell disease	Step-down to CPAP from invasive ventilation 1ˢᵗ 24–48 hours

Table 1.2 *Continued*

	Paediatric High-Dependency Care Unit	Paediatric Intensive Care Unit
2	Exchange transfusion for moderate complications of sickle cell disease	Severe complications of sickle cell crises – e.g. neurological/acute chest
3	Meningococcal septicaemia – stable state – 1st 12–48 hours	Meningococcal septicaemia with shock
4	Diabetic ketoacidosis with drowsiness	Diabetic ketoacidosis with deteriorating level of consciousness after start of therapy, DKA in a child <2 years old
5	Acute renal failure (urine output <1 ml/kg/hour) with serum Potassium ≥5.5 and/or metabolic acidosis	Acute renal support – continuous veno-venous hemofiltration, peritoneal dialysis
6	Moderate metabolic derangement, fluid or electrolyte (Na, K, Ca, Bicarb, Gluc) imbalance requiring cardiac monitoring and without altered sensorium	Severe metabolic derangement, fluid or electrolyte imbalance requiring intensive monitoring or complex interventions or with altered sensorium
7	Toxic ingestion with potential for acute major organ decompensation	Toxic ingestion with acute major organ decompensation
8	Grade 1 hepatic encephalopathy	≥Grade 2 hepatic encephalopathy, ALF with cardiorespiratory instability
9	Acute gastrointestinal bleeding without cardiorespiratory instability	Acute/severe gastrointestinal bleeding with cardiorespiratory instability
10	After high-risk surgery* – triggering PEWT† or requiring closer nursing supervision for potential deterioration despite appropriate management	After high-risk surgery* requiring intensive care support or invasive monitoring
11	Postoperative patients with drain losses >5 ml/kg/hour for >2 hrs; or with active bleeding	Acute organ failure, or established chronic disease with *acute severe* clinical deterioration or secondary failure in another organ – requiring intensive care support
12	Major organ trauma – triggering the PEWT†	Significant/major trauma – requiring intensive care support
13	Deteriorating on PEWT† despite appropriate intervention	Deteriorating on PEWT† despite appropriate intervention

*High-risk surgery – major neurosurgery, major upper airway surgery, major craniofacial surgery, major thoracic surgery, organ transplantation, surgery for thoracic or abdominal trauma, surgery for active gastrointestinal bleeding, surgery with major blood loss, surgery with haemodynamic or respiratory instability – with potential for deterioration despite appropriate postoperative management and requiring frequent monitoring.
†PEWT – Paediatric Early Warning Tool.
As a guide, patients with potentially unstable non-life-threatening moderate disease requiring multidisciplinary intervention, frequent monitoring ± neurological assessment may require consideration for admission to the Paediatric High-Dependency Care Unit.
Patients with severe unstable or life-threatening disease or requiring an intensive-care dependent procedure will require admission to the Paediatric Intensive Care Unit.

Table 1.3 Referral Guidelines for the Paediatric Intensive Care Unit.

E	Paediatric Intensive Care Unit
14	Post-cardiopulmonary resuscitation
15	Electrical or other environmental (e.g. lightning) injuries
16	Suspected or documented malignant hyperthermia
17	Assisted respiration (e.g. bag and mask) or ventilation *other than during recovery from anaesthetic*
18	Recently extubated following prolonged ventilation
19	Newly placed tracheostomy with/without need for mechanical ventilation

I	Intensive-Care Dependent Procedures
1	Endotracheal intubation
2	Endotracheal intubation and mechanical ventilation for acute deterioration, regardless of aetiology
3	Emergency thoracocentesis or pericardiocentesis
4	Inotropic, vasoactive or antiarrhythmic drug infusions
5	Cardioversion, cardiac pacing
6	Mechanical circulatory support
7	Continuous invasive cardiovascular pressure monitoring – central venous or arterial line
8	Induced hypothermia
9	Acute renal support – continuous veno-venous haemofiltration, peritoneal dialysis, plasmafiltration
10	Balloon tamponade of oesophageal varices

Table 1.4 Non-High Dependency and Non-Intensive Care Unit Patients.

S	Ward Care – Specialty Wards and 'Special-ing'
1	Pre- or postoperative patients on appropriate management, IV fluid replacement, requiring analgesic infusion, without respiratory or haemodynamic or CNS compromise, and not triggering PEWT*
2	Hourly drain/nasogastric loss replacement <5 ml/kg/hour
3	Routine post-sedation monitoring
4	Routine post-procedure/post-operation observations
5	Mature stable tracheostomy/stable artificial airway
6	Stable long-term ventilation via stable tracheostomy/face mask
7	Stable or recovering patient requiring $FiO_2 \leq 0.5$ via headbox or facemask to maintain $SaO_2 > 92\%$
8	Acute asthma on $\geq\frac{1}{2}$-hourly nebulizers
9	Diabetic ketoacidosis without altered sensorium
10	Routine neurological observations
11	Head injury without neurological signs
12	Post-seizure monitoring without respiratory or haemodynamic compromise
13	Frequent dressings/suctioning/physiotherapy/positioning
14	Frequent monitoring of blood tests – blood glucose, Hb, INR, U&Es, blood gases, etc.
15	Patient triggering the PEWT[†] but on a stable or improving trend

[†]PEWT – Paediatric Early Warning Tool.

Table 1.5 Discharge and Transfer Guidelines for the Paediatric High-Dependency Care Patient.

Discharge to the general or specialty care paediatric ward
1   Stable respiratory status and airway patency or extubated with evidence of acceptable gas exchange for at least 4 hours
2   FiO$_2$ requirement of ≤ 0.4
3   Stable haemodynamic values for at least 6 hours
4   No requirement of IV inotropes/vasodilators/antiarrhythmic drugs
5   Cardiac arrhythmias controlled for ≥ 24 hours
6   All invasive haemodynamic monitoring devices have been removed
7   Neurological stability with control of seizures for at least 6 hours
8   In chronic disease, resolution of acute illness requiring high dependency/ intensive care with return to baseline clinical status
9   Where decision is made by careful multidisciplinary assessment that course of treatment is medically futile or of no benefit

Note: As a guide, the resolution or stabilization of referring symptoms or physiological condition will indicate readiness for discharge from High Dependency Unit.

Lead centres have the advantage of usually having high dependency and intensive care facilities on site. Staff in district general hospitals are often anxious that their care delivery may be inadequate. In fact necessity means that many nursing staff in district hospitals are highly skilled in the recognition and treatment of children requiring high dependency care, when by definition they perhaps should be transferred to a lead centre. Limited bed availability in lead centres means that only those children who require mechanical ventilation are retrieved and transferred to a lead centre. The Children's Acute Transport Service currently reviews cases on an individual basis as beds allocation is so challenging.

So, with limited beds in lead centres it is paramount that practitioners understand the background of high dependency care and how to optimize care delivery in whatever clinical setting they find themselves in.

Clinical decision-making – why is care suboptimal?

The main theme identified in the literature is that patients admitted from hospital wards to intensive care units (ICU) have a higher overall percentage mortality than patients admitted from other areas of the hospital (Goldhill *et al.* 1999a, 1999b; McGloin *et al.* 1999). In a frequently cited report, McQuillan *et al.* (1998) state that the care of critically ill patients in ward settings, that is, high dependency care, is suboptimal, leading to preventable collapses. The following themes are evident as reasons for this suboptimal care.

Lack of knowledge

Seriously ill patients may be identified by the clinical signs of life-threatening dysfunction of the airway, breathing or circulation, but these may be missed, misinterpreted or mismanaged. The main reasons for this are lack of knowledge and failure to appreciate urgency (McQuillan *et al.* 1998). Respiratory management is the cornerstone of paediatric critical care management and it is possible that early airway management skills may have a profound effect on outcome (Wade 2002). However, evidence demonstrates significant worsening of respiratory rate over the 24 hours before ICU admission and that patients coming to ICU from the wards are often in hospital and seriously ill for some time before ICU admission (Goldhill *et al.* 1999b). Further prospective studies demonstrate that there is a failure in early detection and recognition of patients at risk of acute deterioration (Hillman *et al.* 2001; McArthur Rouse 2001; Coombs and Dillon 2002).

Knowing when to call for assistance

In addition to and probably compounded by a lack of knowledge is the apparent confusion of some ward nurses as to when to summon emergency assistance. The circumstances under which nursing staff contact the emergency team is not well documented (Daffurn *et al.* 1994).

Cioffi's (2000) exploratory study of the experience of nurses summoning emergency assistance demonstrated uncertainty when calling for help due to feelings of 'doing the right thing', 'feeling like an idiot' and 'having a gut feeling'. However, McArthur Rouse (2001) suggests it should not be necessary for registered nurses to require a prompt to call a doctor.

A paediatric nursing audit at King's College Hospital revealed a theory–practice gap, that is, many nurses feel competent to care for high dependency children but also state that they do not have adequate postregistration education in order to care for these patients. The audit figures also represent continued confusion as to when to call for emergency assistance and who should do this.

Communication

Groom (2001) suggests that traditionally, intensive care has been seen as a 'fortress like', 'no go area' where staff are elitist. Coombs and Dillon (2002) states that critical care nurses and ward nurses working alongside each other can enable learning about each other's roles. Critical care nurses need to appreciate the diversity and complexity of the pressures under which acute ward nurses work and not expect unrealistic standards of them (Gibson 1997).

A further barrier to the provision of effective care for the critically ill child is the communication between nurses and doctors. Conflict between nurses and doctors is well documented and commonly referred to as the 'doctor–nurse game' based on the straightforward hierarchical relationship which underpins the roles (Snelgrove and Hughes 2000).

The lived experience of the ward nurse caring for a critically ill child

A hermeneutic study identified the following central themes providing understanding of the lived experience of a ward nurse caring for critically ill children: professional relationships with doctors, the role of intuition, the reflective experience of caring for critically ill children and the caring role of the nurse. In addition to the existing literature these findings serve to bridge the gap between what is familiar in our worlds and what is unfamiliar; we are familiar with nurses in acute ward settings caring for critically ill children but have been unfamiliar with the meaning of this phenomenon (Day 2004).

Understanding of the lived experience of ward nurses caring for critically ill children, personal experience, audit and research and literature findings have facilitated the development of the King's College model (Day *et al.* 2005) (Figure 1.1).

Key objectives of the King's College model

1 To facilitate a multidisciplinary approach for the identification and categorization of high dependency children
2 To facilitate an effective multidisciplinary approach to high dependency provision and the utilization of expert nurses crossing boundaries to enhance continuity of patient care (as advocated by the Department of Health)
3 To identify key personnel required for an effective high dependency service utilizing cost-effective workforce planning strategies
4 To provide evidence of initiatives at King's as a leading teaching hospital to contribute to national initiatives on development of high dependency in paediatrics (nursing)
5 To facilitate collaboration between all departments
6 To improve nursing and retention recruitment strategies.

The implementation of this model demonstrably reduced morbidity on the general wards reflected in a significant reduction in cardiac arrest calls and emergency internal admissions to the paediatric intensive care unit. Advanced nursing practice was recently added to the

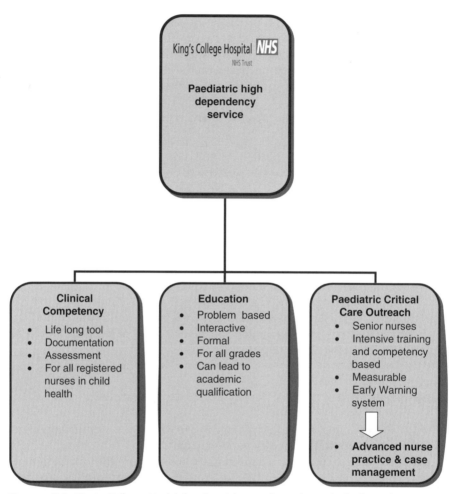

Figure 1.1 King's College Model for the delivery of paediatric high dependency care. Source: Day *et al.* (2005).

model as it was realized that nursing expertise and skills contribute greatly to optimizing the care of critically ill children (Llewellyn and Day 2008).

Components of the model

1. Competency

The Nursing and Midwifery Council has a statutory duty to maintain standards of professional practice and the Code of Professional Conduct

(2008) provides strong guidance to practitioners, thus contributing to the level of competence required for specific activities. However, determining competence is not an easy task. Competence is arguably one of the most commonly used words in education at this point in time but provides a well-recognized dichotomy of theory and practice. It is imperative that a holistic conceptualization of competency is achieved by nurses that empowers practitioners and facilitates critical thinking rather than emphasizing outcome over the importance of the educational process and the use of a variety of forms of knowledge in nursing practice (Milligan 1998).

We recommend, in accordance with practice at King's College Hospital, that all registered nurses, no matter what area they work in, have a comprehensive document that includes, for the first time, level 1 care (high dependency). The document should cover all aspects of clinical care and professional development issues, and provides practitioners with an opportunity to individualize their professional development and career progression. It focuses on the needs of the child and their family and not on the grade of the nurses, thereby ensuring that the family remain at the centre of everything we do and that optimum quality care is delivered at all times. Competency documents can be developed in line with the *Knowledge and Skills Framework* (Department of Health 2004b); then professional development and performance will link directly with mentorship and appraisal.

Common problems associated with competency documentation include lack of time for mentors to complete documents, lack of assessors with appropriate skills in high dependency, managers too busy to ensure the document is implemented, documents are forgotten about if not used and discussed on a regular basis. Strategies to overcome these problems include the development of an assessor's guide to aid completion, utilization of the critical outreach nurse to help complete some of the more complex aspects of the document, and regular audits of the use of the document. An education programme is required to facilitate progression through the document.

2. Education

Evidence of suboptimal care means that the clinical area of critical care has been exposed to both public and political scrutiny (Coombs and Dillon 2002). Two Department of Health documents – *Comprehensive Critical Care: a review of adult critical care services* (2000) and the *National Service Framework for Children, Young People and Maternity Services* (2004a) – have prompted educational initiatives to provide internal and external high dependency education.

The Audit Commission (1999) suggested that ward nurses could not care for higher dependency patients unless they were trained and supported. Nurses themselves have identified the need for continuing educational activities in dealing with acutely and critically ill patients. However, a lack of time, money and appropriate courses often prevents nurses from getting the necessary training.

The impact of continuing professional education in the workplace depends not only on the utility of the knowledge acquired during the course but also on the social context of nursing work, including organizational arrangements and social relationships that affect nurses' ability to apply their new knowledge in practice (Jordan and Hughes 1998).

There are a limited number of recognized course for nurses in high dependency care, there are limited places and timetables are not flexible. To address lack of postregistration education and to support the competency document, an internal structured education programme can be developed and implemented. The aim of the programme should be to teach and for many, consolidate, high dependency skills based on the following principles:

- Clinical assessment skills using a medical model approach
- Recognition of the critically ill child using a problem-based approach
- When to call for assistance
- Referral strategies.

Having a mix of grades and nurses from specialist areas attending the course results in a wealth of experience being shared and examples given, providing opportunity for reflection and problem solving.

3. Paediatric critical care outreach

The use of expert nurses crossing boundaries, or outreach nurses, facilitates empowerment of ward staff by underpinning clinical practice with the knowledge and skills that are necessary to care effectively for the critically ill child. Clinically based practitioners have been identified as the most important role models to help learners translate theory into practice (Coad and Haines 1999).

The Department of Health document *Comprehensive Critical Care: a review of adult critical care services* (2000) called for a hospital-wide approach to the care of critically ill patients. The nursing section of this document states that each critically ill patient, wherever they are located in the hospital, should have skilled critical care nursing available either to care directly for them or to advise on the care required to meet their needs. With this came the establishment of many critical care outreach services in many forms and the use of early warning scoring (EWS).

EWS is the use of a system that utilizes vital signs and urine output to score a patient, providing a means of direction for care in association with clinical examination. EWS has been used in adult nursing in many hospitals and useful literature is available on its effectiveness (Goldhill *et al.* 1999b; Hillman *et al.* 2001; McArthur Rouse 2001). In addition the success of outreach was published in a Department of Health document in 2003, leaving little doubt of its effectiveness. However, little has been documented regarding paediatrics. This is probably due to difficulties in paediatrics due to varying vital signs through age ranges. The aim of the King's College Hospital critical care outreach service is to provide clinical support and critical care skills for the acute ward areas. This is achieved through:

- support for ward staff caring for acutely ill patients who with that support, can safely be managed on a general ward;
- early identification and support of patients requiring intensive care/ high dependency care;
- facilitation of timely admission to intensive care/high dependency care;
- increase in support for patients discharged from intensive care to acute ward areas;
- help in identification of patients for whom intensive care is inappropriate through discussion with relevant clinical teams. In addition, there is evidence that the transfer of a child from the paediatric intensive care unit (PICU) is a stressful experience for parents. Although discharge from PICU is a positive milestone there are associated stresses; adaptation to new staff, a new environment and different approaches to care (Keogh 2001). Critical care outreach facilitates the transition of care from PICU to the ward providing the parents and child with a familiar face and continuity of care.

Preparation

Successful implementation of such a big initiative requires effective communication. The initiative should not be intensive-care dominated as this would prevent the breakdown of barriers between intensive care and the ward areas. Opportunities to discuss and educate all staff should be taken in a multidisciplinary setting. In this way, ward staff feel part of the development team and have some ownership of the process.

Much of the preparation involves development of paperwork and databases that facilitate the utilization of data to assess the effectiveness of outreach, for example, who utilized the service, what outreach nurses were commonly doing on an outreach visit, the number of visits. The final proforma for referral or follow-up can be produced using the ideas suggested by the ward staff during their teaching.

Who can 'outreach'?

A new service should be started using highly experienced nurses with demonstrable paediatric intensive care or high dependency experience with associated qualifications and an advanced life support qualification. In addition, the facilitator of the service should have demonstrable teaching and research and audit experience, relevant postgraduate qualification incorporating advanced clinical assessment skills thus ensuring a service with inbuilt professional accountability for the role.

As the service becomes established and an effective outreach competency document put in place then more staff from other ward areas can be trained in the role and the costs distributed appropriately.

Clinical competence for outreach nurses

The natural progression following the implementation of a comprehensive competency document in paediatrics is to use the same structure to develop a document for outreach nurses. The document should incorporate the core skills for outreach nurses with a focus on clinical examination, teaching and communication. Specific areas are identified as essential or preferable for permanent or seconded team members. Seconded members work with the outreach facilitator until they are confident, completed their competency booklet and have assessed a minimum of six patients under supervision.

Measuring effectiveness

Effectiveness should be measured subjectively with the use of informal feedback methods; the development of an outreach link nurse system provides opportunity for reflection and a forum to present issues, ideas and constructive feedback. Feedback in King's College is that the ward nurses expressed feeling supported rather than a sense of abandonment if a patient is discharged to them from the paediatric intensive care unit. There is a natural increase in clinical teaching and the nursing staff feel more empowered to perform assessment and certain skills knowing they have an experienced practitioner there to support them, for example, care of chest drains, nasopharyngeal suction, choosing oxygen delivery systems. This in turn leads to an increased number of referrals to the outreach team as nurses are recognizing the sick child before the child deteriorates to an uncompensated state.

Early warning systems

An 'early warning system' is a clinical tool that can be used to assess the severity of a patient's illness by reviewing physiological observations in a structured approach.

If the patient's vital signs fall into any of the categories identified by the tool, 'calling criteria' are put into place and consequently a system of timely management of the patient.

Adult scoring systems are well established and supported by the Department of Health, however there are very few validated early warning scores available for children. A choice of system should be made based on local experience and what practitioners regard as user friendly. Some units choose to redesign their observation charts to incorporate the EWS, which allows early recognition of trends and facilitates audit and risk management, rather than adding to an already large amount of paperwork with an additional form. It is also useful to develop posters for key clinical areas to remind practitioners of the appropriate course of action for each trigger or score.

The first system to be validated for children after extensive research was the Bristol tool (Box 1.1). The paediatric critical care outreach practitioner is called when a child triggers any one of the clinical alerts. Another example of an early warning system is that developed in Brighton (Table 1.6). The associated action plan is specific to Brighton but of course can be modified to be used in other paediatric areas. It is not advisable to amend the scores as it is these figures that have been validated for appropriate sensitivity.

Box 1.1 The Bristol Modified Paediatric Early Warning Tool

A Acute airway obstruction
1 Child has required nebulized adrenaline
2 Clinically tiring or impending complete airway obstruction
B Breathing
1 $SaO_2 \leq 92\%$ in any amount of oxygen
2 $SaO_2 \leq 75\%$ in any amount of oxygen (cyanotic heart disease)
3 Persistent tachypnoea (RR ≥ 70 under 6 mo; ≥ 60 6–12 mo, ≥ 40 1–5 yrs, ≥ 25 over 5 yrs)
4 Apnoea +/− bradycardia (HR ≤ 95 in children under 5 yrs)
C Circulation
1 Persistent tachycardia following one bolus of 10 ml/kg fluid (HR ≥ 150 under 5 yrs; HR ≥ 120 5–12 yrs; HR ≥ 100 over 12 yrs)

2 Signs of shock: e.g. prolonged capillary refill time (≥3s); poor perfusion; +/− low BP

D Disability

1 GCS ≤ 11 *or* unresponsive *or* responding only to pain

2 Convulsion unresponsive to anticonvulsant therapy (lasting ≥30 mins)

E Others

1 Hyperkalaemia – K⁺ ≥ 6.0 mmol/l

2 Any child with suspected meningococcus

3 Any child with diabetic ketoacidosis (DKA) with pH < 7 and/or >10% dehydration

4 Any child whose clinical condition is worrying

Source: Haines *et al.* (2006)

Table 1.6 Royal Alexandra Hospital for Sick Children, Brighton Paediatric Early Warning Score. Adapted from Monaghan (2005).

	0	1	2	3	Score
Behaviour	Playing/ appropriate	Sleeping	Irritable	Lethargic/ confused, reduced response to pain	
Cardiovascular	Pink or capillary refill 1–2 s	Pale or capillary refill 3 s	Grey or capillary refill 3 s. Tachycardia of 20 above normal rate	Grey and mottled or capillary refill 5 s or above. Tachycardia of 30 above normal rate or bradycardia	
Respiratory	Within normal parameters, no recession or tracheal tug	>10 above normal parameters, using accessory muscles, 30+% FiO₂ or 4+ litres/min	>20 above normal parameters, recessing, tracheal tug, 40+% FiO₂ or 6+ litres/min	5 below normal parameters with sternal recession, tracheal tug or grunting, 50% FiO₂ or 8+ litres/min	

Score 2 extra for ¼ hourly nebulizers or persistent vomiting following surgery.
Score 2: inform nurse in charge.
Score 3: increase frequency of score and observations using outreach observation chart, and inform nurse in charge.
Score 4 or if score increases by 2 following interventions: call medical staff and inform outreach coordinator. Medical staff should respond in 15 minutes.
Score >4 or any red column: immediately call senior registrar, anaesthetist and outreach coordinator. Consider transfer.

Issues to consider when setting up a high dependency service

There are some key issues that need to be considered when setting up a high dependency service in a paediatric department. These can be divided into the following categories:

- location
- equipment
- staffing
- resources
- education.

Some of these issues have been covered already in this chapter and these will not be discussed again, but some issues warrant further examination.

Location

The location of a high dependency service is key both to the ability of the unit to effectively staff the service and for the safety of the patients. Issues that need to be considered when deciding on the location include the closeness of the area to the nurse's station if you have one, the physical size of the area and the physical resources available in the area such as piped oxygen and suction. Proximity to other staff members is important as it allows staff working in the high dependency area to be able to call on other staff members in a crisis and it also allows easy cover for staff rest breaks. The physical size of the area is crucial, as children requiring high dependency care often have a lot of equipment around their bed space and it is important to provide enough space for this and also for staff to attend to the patient easily. Parental presence will also need to be considered, particularly at night time, so providing adequate space for a parent to both sit and rest is important.

The area also needs to have the correct services such as piped oxygen, air and suction. If the intention is to provide short-term ventilation then piped air is essential for this and is not always available on normal ward areas. It is also much better for monitoring equipment to be placed on the walls as permanent fixtures rather than on the top of lockers or trolleys.

If it is not possible for a particular area to be designated for high dependency care then the Department of Health (2002) recommends that as a minimum an area is available for resuscitation and a mobile trolley with the necessary equipment is ready at all times to be moved to the location where it is required.

Equipment

Providing a high dependency service requires a capital investment. The Department of Health (2001) recommends that the following equipment is provided as a minimum:

- Piped medical gases and suction
- Multi-module monitor to include ECG, respiration, invasive and noninvasive pressure monitoring, end tidal CO_2, temperature, pulse oximetry
- Hand ventilation circuit
- Syringe pumps
- Infusion pumps
- Suction unit
- Oxygen analyser.

Some equipment does not need to be provided in the high dependency area itself but needs to be readily available:

- Defibrillator
- Resuscitation trolley
- Thermal care centre
- Equipment for providing oxygen therapy
- Blood gas analysis equipment
- CPAP driver and anaesthetic machine.

If the high dependency unit is to be located in a district general hospital then there may need to be some disposable equipment available that would not normally be used. This would include:

- Central venous pressure lines
- Arterial lines
- Chest drains
- Circuits for ventilators and CPAP machines
- Transducer sets for invasive pressure monitoring.

It is important that staff have the regular opportunity to handle and set up unfamiliar equipment so that they feel confident to use it should the need arise. Regular updating sessions should form part of the continuing education programme for all staff.

Staffing

Having appropriately qualified staff is essential for providing a safe and effective high dependency service. A lead clinician for high dependency should be identified in all hospitals treating children (Department of Health 2001) and a member of medical staff with the appropriate paediatric advanced life support certification should be available 24 hours a day. The lead clinician is responsible for planning and overseeing the service and developing links with the local paediatric intensive care service to enable them to provide support to the hospital.

Staff ratios are identified in relation to the patient's level of dependency. At least one member of nursing staff working in the area must as a minimum have received the appropriate training in advanced paediatric life support (Department of Health 2001). As already mentioned, there are a few recognized high dependency courses for nursing staff but they are dependent upon local provision.

Resources

Appropriate financial and physical resources will need to be provided if a high dependency service is to be run effectively and safely. All units providing high dependency care should have a system of clinical audit and governance to ensure that care is provided optimally at all times. For staff unfamiliar with running a high dependency service or if the providing of high dependency care is not a regular occurrence, then an integrated care pathway (ICP) may provide a system that ensures appropriate care is provided. An ICP is a multidisciplinary outline of anticipated care which helps a patient with a specific condition or set of symptoms move through a clinical experience (Middleton *et al.* 2001). Using ICPs may help to standardize care and provide a structure for staff to follow.

Conclusion

Paediatric high dependency provision presents a significant clinical challenge. Defining and understanding the meaning of high dependency care goes some way in optimizing care. The King's College model provides a framework of clinical competency, education and critical care outreach, and early data suggests the model is effective in improving care and contributes to maintaining high quality care.

Learning activities

- Reflect on a situation where you have had to provide high dependency care. Did any of the factors described in 'Clinical decision making' occur? What would you do differently in a similar situation?
- Write a clinical scenario that and care plan for a 3-year-old with acute asthma over a time period of 3 hours. Consider potential issues in the delivery of high dependency care in your workplace including skills and manpower and the potential use of an early warning system.
- Formulate a discussion on the potential difficulties of arranging the transfer of a child requiring high dependency care to a lead centre. Consider practical problems, clinical risk, manpower and the family.

References and further reading

Audit Commission (1999) *Critical to Success*. Audit Commission, London.

Coad S, Haines S (1999) Supporting staff caring for critically ill patients in acute ward areas. *Nursing in Critical Care* 4(5): 245–249.

Cioffi J (2000) Nurses' experiences of making decisions to call emergency assistance to their patients. *Journal of Advanced Nursing* 32(1): 108–114.

Coombs M, Dillon A (2002) Crossing boundaries, re defining care: the role of the critical care outreach team. *Journal of Clinical Nursing* 11(3): 387–393.

Daffurn K, Lee A, Hillman KM, Bishop GF, Bauman A (1994) Do nurses know when to summon emergency assistance? *Intensive and Critical Care Nursing* 10: 115–120.

Day H (2004) Exploring the meaning of caring for a critically ill child on the general paediatric ward. City University London (unpublished).

Day H, Allen Z, Llewellyn L (2005) The development of a paediatric high dependency service. *Paediatric Nursing* 17(3): 24–28.

Department of Health (1997) *Paediatric Intensive Care: a framework for the future*. DH, London.

Department of Health (2000) *Comprehensive Critical Care: a review of adult critical care services*. DH, London.

Department of Health (2001) Setting up high dependency service???

Department of Health (2002) *High Dependency Care for Children* – Report of an expert advisory group. DH, London.

Department of Health (2003) *Critical Care Outreach – Progress in developing services*. DH, London.

Department of Health (2004a) *National Service Framework for Children, Young People and Maternity Services.* DH, London.

Department of Health (2004b) *The NHS Knowledge Skills Framework.* DH, London.

Gibson JME (1997) Focus of nursing in critical and acute care settings: prevention or cure? *Intensive and Critical Care Nursing* **13**: 163–166.

Goldhill DR, Worthington L, Mulcahy A, Tarling M, Sumner A (1999a) The patient at risk team: identifying and managing seriously ill ward patients. *Anaesthesia* **54**: 853–860.

Goldhill D, White S, Sumner A (1999b) Physiological values and procedures in the 24h before ICU admission form the ward. *Anaesthesia* **54**: 529–34.

Groom P (2001) Critical care outreach teams – a prayer answered? *Nursing Times* **97**(43): 34.

Hillman K, Parr M, Flabouris A, Bishop G, Stewart A (2001) Redefining in hospital resuscitation: the concept of the medical emergency team. *Resuscitation* **48**: 105–110.

Jordan S, Hughes D (1998) Using bioscience knowledge in nursing: actions, interactions and reactions. *Journal of Advanced Nursing* **27**: 1060–1068.

Keogh S (2001) Parent's experience of the transfer of their child from PICU to the ward: a phenomenological study. *Nursing in Critical Care* **6**(1): 7–13.

Llewellyn L, Day H (2008) Advancing nursing practice in paediatric critical care. *Paediatric Nursing* **20**(1): 30–33.

McArthur Rouse F (2001) Critical care outreach services and early warning scoring systems: a review of the literature. *Journal of Advanced Nursing* **36**(5): 696–704.

McGloin H, Adam S, Singer M (1999) Unexpected deaths and referrals to intensive care of patents on general wards. Are some cases potentially avoidable? *Journal of the Royal College of Physicians of London* **33**(3): 255–259.

McQuillan P, Pilkington S, Allan A, *et al.* (1998) Confidential inquiry into the quality of care before admission to intensive care. *British Medical Journal* **316**: 1853–1858.

Middleton S, Barnett J, Reeves D (2001) What is an integrated care pathway? www.evidence-based-medicine.co.uk. Hayward Medical Publications.

Milligan F (1998) Defining and assessing competence. *Nurse Education Today* **18**: 273–280.

Monaghan A (2005) Detecting and managing deterioration in children. *Paediatric Nursing* **17**(1) 32–35.

Nursing and Midwifery Council (2008) *Code of Professional Conduct* 2008.

PICS Standards document (2001) *Referral to the Paediatric Intensive Care Unit.*

Snelgrove S, Hughes D (2000) Interprofessional relations between doctors and nurses: perspectives from South Wales. *Journal of Advanced Nursing* **31**(3): 661–667.

Tume L (2007) The deterioration of children in ward areas in a specialist children's hospital. *Nursing in Critical Care* **12**(1): 12–19.

Wade K (2002) Paediatric high dependency provision a case for urgent review ion the United Kingdom. *Intensive and Critical Care Nursing* **18**: 109–117.

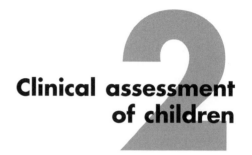

Clinical assessment of children

Helen Day and Andrea Cockett

Learning outcomes

- To develop an understanding of the stages of clinical assessment
- To develop an understanding of the classifications and recognition of shock

Introduction

The aim of this chapter is to provide the knowledge you require to perform a structured and rapid clinical assessment. This is paramount when caring for children in the high dependency setting as it enables you to gain all the relevant clinical information to facilitate nursing care and treatment. The findings of an effective clinical assessment allow recognition and treatment of potential respiratory, cardiovascular or neurological failure. In addition, an experienced practitioner will also be considering specific clinical possibilities within a given specialty to explain clinical deterioration or changes in condition; subsequent chapters will highlight these specialist findings. The presentation and treatment of shock is also explained in this chapter, as early recognition of shock is vital to prevent rapid deterioration within any clinical specialty.

It is vital that appropriate mentorship is provided in your workplace and you can practise your assessments under supervision until deemed competent in accordance with your local guidelines.

Practitioners wishing to advance their practice should refer to texts describing full medical examination. This chapter aims to provide an overview of the five components of clinical assessment to guide your practice within a high dependency setting.

Rapid assessment

Regardless of specialty, if you suspect serious deterioration an 'AVPU' and 'ABC' approach should be adopted immediately.

AVPU

A: Alert

V: Voice
Patient only responding to voice – Glasgow Coma Scale (GCS) equivalent 11. Obtain medical assistance quickly and continue with your clinical assessment and interventions.

P: Pain
Patient only responsive to pain – GCS equivalent 8. Obtain medical assistance immediately. A GCS of 8 indicates potential airway compromise. Continue with your clinical assessment.

U: Unresponsive
A patient who is unresponsive but breathing has an equivalent GCS of 3 and is at the stage of imminent cardiorespiratory arrest. A cardiac arrest call should be made.

Remember
Interventions for all high dependency children in assessment phase: oxygen and monitoring

ABC

If the patient is not breathing then life support should be commenced using an airway, breathing, circulation (ABC) approach as per UK Resuscitation Council guidelines:

1. SAFE approach (SAFE: Shout for help, Approach with care, Free from danger, Evaluate ABC)
2. Airway opening manoeuvres
3. Look, listen, feel for breathing
4. Commence bag valve mask ventilations '5 rescue breaths'
5. Check pulse and signs of circulation
6. CPR: 12 chest compressions: 2 ventilations
7. Commence advanced life support procedures when assistance arrives.

If you are satisfied that your patient is stable, utilize a structured approach to continue clinical assessment.

Structured clinical assessment

Components of clinical assessment

Standard precautions during clinical assessment of all patients:

*   Wash hands
*   Wear apron
*   Wear gloves if risk of contact with bodily fluids
*   Take care with linen
*   Ensure privacy
*   Explanations to patient or parents where necessary.

History
A full medical history should be taken by the appropriate practitioner, and indeed may have already have been taken if the child has deteriorated in hospital. However, in the high dependency setting 'the history' is usually narrowed down to the child's current problem. All the information should be put together with the findings of physical examination to facilitate clinical decision-making. In the high dependency setting it is useful to take a history following a system approach:

*   Reason for admission to high dependency unit? Presenting symptoms:
    *   respiratory: including interventions, and effectiveness
    *   cardiovascular including interventions and effectiveness
    *   neurological

- abdominal/gastrointestinal, liver
- renal.

Even in the case of a potentially critically ill child, history and information from the child and parents will be useful, though this may not always be easy to obtain. Dependent on the age, severity of illness and cognitive development stage of the child, accurate information may be almost impossible to obtain from the child directly. However this does not mean you simply ignore the child. Any information will be valuable and children may have a valuable contribution to be made and want to give it. A general rule is that children over 5 will give a fairly accurate account of how they are feeling but it may be the information gained from the parent or guardian that is more accurate. Parents are often distressed and anxious. Allow them time to calm down and perhaps take this opportunity to perform your physical assessment while giving thorough explanations of what you are doing to both the parent or guardian and the child if appropriate. This may be a good time to introduce the play specialist who is an invaluable member of the team throughout the patient stay, using expert distraction and therapeutic play techniques to facilitate optimum treatment and recovery.

Taking a full history may not always be relevant unless you have a new patient, but always check to see that a thorough history has been taken and, if in doubt of any details, take it again. If you are working in a high dependency unit and the child is being transferred to you from a general ward setting, take time to listen to the ward staff handover as it will provide you with an accurate picture of recent clinical events. It is all too easy to get wrapped up in the here and now and to miss key details from the previous few hours.

Although history is conveniently the first step in your assessment process it must never be at the expense of necessary clinical intervention. If appropriate, perform your physical assessment first, intervene as appropriate, reassess and come back to the history. A skilled practitioner will be able to ask pertinent questions while performing the physical assessment.

> ## Remember
> Always listen to parents, even those seemingly ill educated may have a remarkable amount of insight. They may not know what is wrong but they will know that something is wrong.

Inspection

Inspection yields the most valuable information during your assessment and the power of observation is the practitioner's greatest skill. Subsequent chapters will address what is entailed in the inspection segment of clinical assessment within that specialty where relevant. This chapter presents the general survey.

It may sound obvious but as you walk towards a patient, observe the immediate physical environment. A child sat up in bed watching television does not give cause for concern but a child who has two intravenous infusions in situ, an obvious wound drain hanging from the bed, a nasogastric tube and a urinary catheter in situ, watching television, should cause you concern. This is because of a very important word in high dependency care: *'potential'*. Recognition of potential problems or deterioration is key to the management of the high dependency child so never take the term 'stable' for granted.

Gill and O'Brien (2003) liken examining children to veterinary medicine.

- Veterinary paediatrics – some attributes shared by animals and small children:
  - They don't like being stared at
  - They lie down when sick
  - Repeated food refusal is unusual
  - They have limited ability to express themselves
  - They adopt the position of comfort when well
  - Their survival instinct is strong.

Theses are indeed useful and humorous tips and can assist with examination of the child:

- Skin: pale? cyanosed? sweating? jaundiced?
- Nails: colour? contour?
- Mouth and tongue
- Demeanour: facial expression? grimace? smile? Dependent on age, is the child making eye contact? Are the eyes open? Is a baby seeking out eye contact with a parent?
- Dependent on age, assess mobility: is the patient mobile? normal gait and balance?
- Nasogastric tube in situ? Spiggoted or on free drainage? What is it draining? Enteral feed pump in situ? Intravenous infusion in situ? Emesis basins visible? Wound drain in situ? What is in the drain?
- Nutritional and hydration status: oedema?
- What position is the patient in? Rigid with pain? Knees up to the abdomen indicating pain? Keeping very still in the bed, indicating pain? Moving freely? Crying without any stimulation?

- Abnormal movements: twitching? shivering?
- Abnormal odours: ketosis? wound infection?

Auscultation

Auscultation is the skill of using a stethoscope. It is also vital to mention that sounds audible without the use of a stethoscope are of great importance and fall in this section of assessment, for example respiratory wheeze.

The *stethoscope* (from Greek, *stéthos* – chest and *skopé* – examination) is an acoustic medical device for auscultation, or listening to, internal sounds in a human or animal body. It is most often used to listen to heart sounds and breathing. It is also used to listen to intestines and blood flow in arteries and veins.

Acoustic stethoscopes are familiar to most people, and work by transmitting sound from the chestpiece, via air-filled hollow tubes, to the listener's ears. The chestpiece usually consists of two sides that can be placed against the patient for sensing sound – a diaphragm (plastic disc) or bell (hollow cup). If the diaphragm is placed on the patient, body sounds vibrate the diaphragm, creating acoustic pressure waves which travel up the tubing to the listener's ears. If the bell is placed on the patient, the vibrations of the skin directly produce acoustic pressure waves travelling up to the listener's ears. The bell transmits low-frequency sounds while the diaphragm transmits higher-frequency sounds.

A stethoscope has traditionally been seen as the doctor's tool. However, while diagnosis may not be within the remit of the nurse it is imperative that nurses have the minimum skill to auscultate the heart and lungs to identify abnormal or extra sounds.

Palpation

Palpation is used as part of a physical examination in which an object is felt (usually with the hands of a healthcare practitioner) to determine its size, shape, firmness, or location. Palpation is typically used for thoracic and abdominal examinations, but can also be used to diagnose oedema and to measure the pulse. Palpation can be divided into light, deep, and palpation during respiration. Again use of palpation as part of an assessment has traditionally been seen as a doctor's role, but a nurse should be able to perform light palpation of the abdomen (see Chapter 7) and be competent in palpating the thoracic area during a respiratory and cardiovascular examination (Chapters 4 and 5), taking all pulses and lastly the blood pressure (see Chapter 3).

Percussion

Percussion is a method of tapping on a surface to determine the under-lying structure, and is used in clinical examinations to assess the condition of the thorax or abdomen It is done with the middle finger of the right hand tapping on the middle finger of the left hand, while the left palm is on the body. Further details are beyond the scope of this book but should be sought if considering advancing nursing practice.

Normal findings:

- Abdomen – tympanic (dull over liver);
- Lungs – resonant (dullness over cardiac borders).

Tip

Once you have completed your clinical assessment, use all the information you have gathered to plan and prioritize your care of the sick child.

Communicating with children and their families

Communication is an essential part of any clinical assessment (Wales *et al.* 2008) it is of particular importance when the child is very unwell and clinical interventions may be occurring at a rapid pace. Families expect clear information on diagnosis, treatment and prognosis (Hummelinck and Pollock 2006). They also expect to participate in the decision-making process that occurs during treatment and interventions (Flatman 2002). It is important that all healthcare professionals involved in the care of the child and family have the appropriate communication skills. Important points to consider when communicating with children include:

- Use the child's age as a starting point to predict their understanding of what is happening to them.
- Offer the child information in a way that will match their level of understanding.
- Be aware of the physical environment and how this will affect the child's understanding and responses.
- Constantly check the child's level of understanding as you are undertaking the assessment.
- Try to use a mixture of open and closed questions. When time is tight and the child's condition is poor you may need to ask closed,

simple-answer questions so that you can undertake the assessment rapidly.

- Be aware of language and cultural issues that may affect the communication process.
- Use play as a way of gaining information form young children.
- Be truthful with the child; the older child will realize that their carers are anxious and this may worry them.

Providing care that is 'family centred' is an important part of any service. Smith *et al.* (2002) define family-centred care as care which is the professional support of the child and family through a process of involvement, participation and partnership, underpinned by empowerment and negotiation. The *National Service Framework for Children, Young People and Maternity Services* (Department of Health 2004) reinforces the importance of family-centred care by stating that services should be coordinated around the child's individual needs as well as the families and take account of their views.

Providing this type of service where children are very ill can be challenging. It can be difficult for parents to participate in care when their child is very unwell as they may be unable to undertake some of the normal caring roles they may fill, but also the medicalization of the care required may leave them feeling inadequate (Haines and Wolstenholme 2000). This is where negotiation becomes a very important part of the parent–practitioner relationship. It is very important that parents feel able to participate in their child's care if they wish, and also that they just support their child emotionally if this is all they feel able to do. The key to providing care for children and families in this situation is to negotiate clearly and frequently with them about what they wish to do and what the treatment involves. For many parents, encouraging them to talk to and touch their child can them help them to go on and take a more active role in the care of their child.

One difficulty that has been identified in relation to high dependency care is the anxiety that parents can feel when their child is transferred from an intensive care environment to a high dependency one (Keogh 2001). The difference in staff to child ratios can cause parents to become very anxious that their child is not receiving the care that they require. They also feel anxious over the amount of monitoring their child may be receiving. Similar feelings may be experienced by parents whose child is transferred from a tertiary centre back to a local hospital. It is very important that parents are prepared adequately for this transfer and that staff are aware of and sensitive to the concerns of parents. What should be a time of reduced anxiety as their child's condition improves can in fact be a time of high stress for many parents. Communication is essential in these situations.

Retrieval of children

Some children receiving high dependency care will need to be transferred to a paediatric intensive care unit if their condition deteriorates. It is now accepted practice that the best way to achieve this transfer is through the use of a retrieval team (Paediatric Intensive Care Society 2001). This ensures that the child is cared for appropriately through the most dangerous part of the procedure, the actual transfer itself. Retrieval of children to tertiary centres is now well established in the United Kingdom and there are well-set-out referral procedures. Retrieval teams are identified for each region and link into the appropriate paediatric intensive care units. Guidance on referral and procedures are available on the web pages of the tertiary centre concerned. Parents will need to be prepared appropriately for the transfer and also for the move to a tertiary service. This may be difficult for them if the distances involved are large and they have other children to care for. It is important that the referring hospital provide the parents with the correct information during what is a very stressful time (Stack and Dobbs 2004).

Shock

Early recognition and treatment of a child in shock is vital to prevent rapid deterioration. Shock is included in this chapter as it is a condition that can present within any specialty and the treatment is the same. The word 'shock' may instil panic into most practitioners; however, with a structured approach and the use of an early warning system, shock can be easily recognized and treated.

What is shock?

Shock is inadequate tissue perfusion resulting in impaired cellular respiration. Shock results from an acute failure of circulatory function and there are five types – hypovolaemia, distributive, cardiogenic, obstructive or dissociative – with the most common in children being hypovolaemic and distributive shock.

Before we go on to define and describe the specific types of shock (see Table 2.1) it is vital to recognize that shock is a progressive syndrome and is conveniently divided into three phases.

Phase 1: Compensated shock
Vital organ function is preserved by sympathetic reflexes, therefore systolic blood pressure remains normal but the key signs we observe

Table 2.1 Classifications of shock.

Type of shock	Examples	Specific clinical signs	Specific clinical treatment
• Hypovolaemic Fluid loss	• Haemorrhage • Gastroenteritis • Intussusception • Volvulus • Burns • Peritonitis	• Increased effort of breathing • Increased heart rate with thready peripheral pulse volume • Delayed capillary refill time	• Oxygen • Fluid bolus, reassess, fluid bolus • Urinary catheter
• Distributive Abnormalities of vessels	• Septicaemia • Anaphylaxis • Vasodilating drugs • Spinal cord injury	• Vasodilation and high cardiac output may cause warm peripheries which should not lull you into false sense of security as it will also be associated with: • Increased heart rate • Increased effort of breathing • Pyrexia • Mental confusion	• Oxygen • Fluid bolus – may need to be reassessed and repeated several times. Hypotension is a poor prognostic indicator and requires emergency and expert help • Treat anaphylaxis appropriately
• Cardiogenic Defects of the pump	• Arrhythmias • Cardiomyopathy • Heart failure • Valvular disease • Myocardial contusion	• Cyanosis not correcting with oxygen therapy • Tachycardia out of proportion to respiratory difficulty • Raised jugular venous pressure • Gallop rhythm • Murmur • Enlarged liver • Absent femoral pulses	• If there is no improvement after oxygen and fluid and any of the specific clinical signs listed are present, refer for expert cardiology help • See chapter 5

Table 2.1 *Continued*

Type of shock	Examples	Specific clinical signs	Specific clinical treatment
• Obstructive	• Tension pnuemothorax • Haemopneumothorax • Flail chest • Cardiac tamponade • Pulmonary embolism	• Have high index of suspicion when a patient has sustained traumatic injuries for: • Tension pneumothorax: respiratory distress, hyper-resonant on affected side, tracheal deviation away from affected side, hypoxic and shocked • Haemothorax: Dullness to percussion, shocked • Flail chest: paradoxical chest movement may be seen, hypoxia despite oxygen, pain • Cardiac tamponade: hypotension, distended neck veins • Pulmonary embolism rare in children	• High flow oxygen for all • Needle decompression for tension pneumothorax • Volume replacement then chest drain for haemothorax • Flail chest; pain relief and oxygen, may need positive pressure ventilation if severely compromised to facilitate unison of floating signet with rest of chest wall • Cardiac tamponade; pericardiocentesis
• Dissociative	• Profound anaemia • Carbon monoxide poisoning • Methaemoglobinaemia	• Carbon monoxide: headache, confusion, coma if untreated • Methaemoglobinaemia; cyanosis	• Anaemia: referral to specialist • Carbon monoxide: high flow oxygen and referral to hyperbaric unit if severely compromised • Methaemoglobinaemia: confirm origin (acquired or congenital). Both respond to methylene blue

are increased heart rate, mild agitation or confusion, and cold peripheries. Tachycardia is frequently ignored or an alternative explanation for its cause given. Tachycardia is a key sign of compensated shock and healthcare practitioners should be acting at this stage to prevent deterioration.

Phase 2: Uncompensated shock
The circulatory system is no longer efficient and anaerobic metabolism becomes the major source of energy production, producing lactate which results in a metabolic acidosis. Anaerobic metabolism and acidosis impair the homeostatic environment in which all cells function. Cascading metabolic changes reduce tissue perfusion and oxidation even further. Clinical signs will be tachycardia, falling blood pressure, tachypnoea, cold peripheries, depressed cerebral state and absent urine output.

Phase 3: Irreversible shock
This diagnosis is retrospective. Damage to key organs is so profound that death occurs despite adequate restoration of the circulation.

Remember

Approach all children using the AVPU and ABC approach until you are satisfied the child is stable and you can move on to your structured examination

---

Remember

Interventions for all high dependency children in assessment phase: oxygen and monitoring

---

Most practitioners have the recognition and treatment of hypovolaemic shock entrenched from an early stage in their careers, but it is only in recent years that that an understanding of the progression of infection to septicaemia and septic shock has come about.

The main clinical differences can be summarized as follows:

- *Hypovolaemic shock* – low intravascular volume, low cardiac output, high vascular resistance, cold peripheries, thready pulse, delayed capillary refill time, narrow pulse pressure.
- *Septic shock* – high cardiac output, low vascular resistance, warm peripheries, bounding pulse, delayed, normal or brisk capillary refill time.

It is easy to take an apparently simple pyrexia for granted, in the belief that paracetamol and antibiotics will cure all. The simple and potential rapid progression from infection to death is represented in Figure 2.1, emphasizing the need for effective recognition and prompt treatment.

Use a structured approach in your assessment and management of a child in shock. In the hospital setting shock should be identified in the compensated stage and early treatment should prevent deterioration and death.

Remember

Always investigate and act on an increased heart rate, increased respiratory rate or altered level of consciousness, no matter how stable or well the patient appears

---

Conclusion

This chapter has provided an overview of clinical assessment for the high dependency patient. The practitioner must make a decision when approaching the patient, as to whether a rapid assessment and resuscitation is required, or whether a structured system review should be performed to facilitate care planning. Shock can occur in any patient within any specialty and should be identified in the compensated stage. Pain is a common occurrence for many patients but should be recognized and treated promptly. The skills for clinical assessment and the identification of shock should now guide you through the remaining specialist chapters.

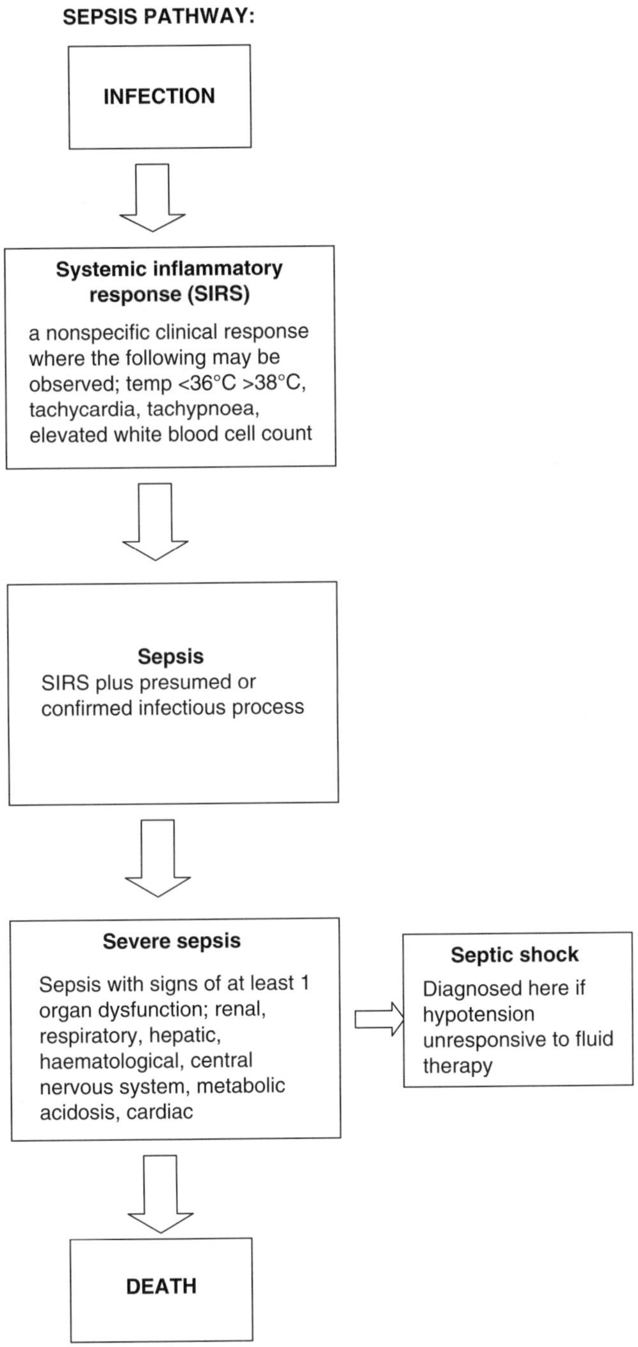

SEPSIS PATHWAY:

INFECTION

⇩

Systemic inflammatory response (SIRS)

a nonspecific clinical response where the following may be observed; temp <36°C >38°C, tachycardia, tachypnoea, elevated white blood cell count

⇩

Sepsis
SIRS plus presumed or confirmed infectious process

⇩

Severe sepsis

Sepsis with signs of at least 1 organ dysfunction; renal, respiratory, hepatic, haematological, central nervous system, metabolic acidosis, cardiac

⇨ **Septic shock**

Diagnosed here if hypotension unresponsive to fluid therapy

⇩

DEATH

Figure 2.1 Progression of sepsis.

Learning activities

- Make time to accompany a nurse practitioner or doctor when they are performing a full clinical exanimation. Identify the process described above. Take note of individuals' helpful tips learnt from experience!
- Take an observation position during a clinical examination following an acute admission. Imagine yourself as a parent and reflect on what can be done to optimize the care and communication of the child and family.
- Ask your mentor to borrow a resuscitation mannequin or ask the resuscitation officer where you work to spend half an hour running through some potential scenarios of children in shock.

References and further reading

Department of Health (2004) *National Service Framework for Children, Young People and Maternity Services.* HMSO, London.

Flatman D (2002) Consulting children: Are we listening? *Paediatric Nursing* **14**(7): 28–31.

Gill D, O'Brien N (2003) *Paediatric Clinical Examination Made Easy.* 4th Edition. Churchill Livingstone, Edinburgh.

Haines C, Wolstenholme M (2000) Family support in paediatric intensive care. In Williams C, Asquith J, *Paediatric Intensive Care Nursing.* Churchill Livingstone, Edinburgh.

Hummelinck A, Pollock K (2006) Parents' information needs about the treatment of their chronically ill child: a qualitative study. *Patient Education and Counselling* **62**(2): 228–234.

Keogh S (2001) Parents' experience of the transfer of their child from PICU to the ward: a phenomenological study. *Nursing in Critical Care* **6**(1): 7–13.

Paediatric Intensive Care Society (2001) *Standards for Paediatric Intensive Care,* 2nd Edition. PICS, Sheffield.

Smith L, Coleman V, Bradshaw M (2002) *Family Centred Care: concept, theory and practice.* Palgrave Macmillan, Basingstoke.

Stack C, Dobbs P (2004) *Essentials of Paediatric Intensive Care.* Greenwich Medical Media, London.

Wales S, Crisp J, Moran P, Perrin M, Scott E (2008) Assessing communication between health professionals, children and families. *Journal of Children and Young People's Nursing* **2**(2): 77–83.

3

Therapeutic interventions for children requiring high dependency care

Leanne Burns

Learning outcomes

- To develop an understanding of the different therapeutic interventions that may be used for children requiring high dependency care
- To develop an understanding of the nursing care for children receiving these interventions

Introduction

The aim of this chapter is to provide an overview of therapeutic interventions a child receiving high dependency care may require. Some of the interventions discussed in this chapter are also covered in other chapters; this is to ensure that the interventions are linked with the disease processes for a specific condition. These children can present with a variety of clinical conditions which may require continuous monitoring to facilitate recognition of changes in their condition and the instigation of early interventions. Nursing observation is the gold standard assessment tool; in addition there are many devices that can aid early recognition of the clinical symptoms which these children may demonstrate, associated with changes in clinical condition. This chapter will consider some of the commonly used monitoring devices in the high dependency unit and provide the reader with insight into indications and appropriate applications.

Blood pressure monitoring

Blood pressure (BP) is the force exerted by circulating blood on the walls of blood vessels (Tortora and Grabowski 1996). The systolic arterial pressure is defined as the peak pressure in the arteries, which occurs near the beginning of the cardiac cycle. The diastolic arterial pressure is the lowest (resting phase) of the cardiac cycle. The average pressure throughout the cardiac cycle is referred to as mean arterial pressure or MAP (Garretson 2005). The unit of measurement for blood pressure is mmHg (Table 3.1).

There are several ways to measure blood pressure in children within the high dependency unit. These are:

- Using a stethoscope and sphygmomanometer;
- Using an automated device that measures pressure non invasively using a cuff;
- Invasive measurement utilizing an intra-arterial line that provides continuous reading.

The speed and reliability of readings from automated devices, together with the hazards of mercury, have made sphygmomanometers almost obsolete in clinical practice (Jones *et al.* 2003). The decision whether to use invasive or non-invasive blood pressure monitoring will depend on the acuity of the child as well as the experience of staff and the environment in which the child is to be nursed (Torrance and Semple 1997).

Measurement of non-invasive blood pressure involves an electronic pressure sensor fitted to detect blood flow. The cuff is inflated and

Table 3.1 Normal values for vital signs.

Age	Systolic BP (mmHg)	Diastolic BP (mmHg)	Mean BP (mmHg)
Newborn (3 kg)	50–70	25–24	40–60
Infant	85–105	55–65	50–90
Toddler	95–105	55–65	50–100
Preschool	95–110	55–65	50–100
School age	95–110	55–70	60–90
Adolescent	110–130	65–80	65–95

released by an electrically operated pump and valve. The cuff is inflated to a pressure initially in excess of the systolic arterial pressure and then reduced to a pressure below diastolic pressure over a period of about 30 seconds. Numerous factors can influence blood pressure including anxiety, pain, position of patient and excursion (Torrance and Semple 1997). The nurse should take this into consideration when interpreting the readings from blood pressure measurement and try to create an environment that limits these factors influencing the reading (e.g. distraction therapies, asking parents to assist, familiarizing the child with the equipment to be used).

If using a non-invasive technique of blood pressure measurement there are several factors that should be taken into consideration.

- Cuff width: the European standard recommends that the length of the cuff bladder be at least 80% of the limb circumference utilized for blood pressure measurement, with the width being a minimum of 40% of the limb (British Hypertension Society 2006). If this is too narrow the blood pressure reading will be falsely high, while a cuff too wide will produce a falsely low reading (British Hypertension Society 2006).
- Position of the arm: the arm should be in a horizontal position at the level of the heart (O'Brien et al 1995). Incorrect positioning of the limb can cause errors of as much as 10% (Jevon and Ewens 2007). To achieve this when measuring a child's blood pressure, the nurse may have to utilize a table with height adjustment or a soft pillow on which the child's arm can be placed.

Complications of non-invasive blood pressure measurement are rare but include limb oedema, friction blisters and compression injury to the ulna nerve (Lodato 1998). It is important to consider that, within the high dependency context, children may have neurological deficit, have received sedation or have possible weakness and therefore their response to such complications may be impaired. It is common practice within high dependency units to change the cuff position 4 hourly with observation of cuff sites done at this time also.

Invasive direct measurement of arterial pressure using an indwelling catheter is generally considered to be the 'gold standard' by which other methods should be judged (Reeves 1995). This method provides second-by-second data, often associated with concern surrounding cardiovascular stability of the child (Garretson 2005).

Common insertion sites for arterial lines in children include:

- radial artery
- femoral artery
- dorsalis pedis artery (foot)

- brachial artery (used less commonly)
- anxilla artery (used less commonly).

The radial and femoral arteries are those most commonly seen in practice. The radial artery is frequently used due to it being easily accessible, in a superficial position and easy to monitor and observe in practice (Hinds and Watson 1999). The brachial and anxilla arteries are used infrequently in children due to complications with tissue perfusion to the lower extremity. Clinicians should evaluate the acuity of the child when determining the need for placement of an arterial line, regardless of the position of insertion.

The patency of the arterial line is paramount if accurate blood pressure monitoring is to be achieved. In practice, patency is maintained by utilizing a pressurized flush bag (Campbell 1997). The flush bag used will vary dependent upon unit protocol. Common practice is to use 500 ml 0.9% saline containing 500 iu heparin, giving a 1 iu heparin/ml solution, although it has been suggested that the removal of heparin from this solution has no adverse affects on arterial line patency (Gamby and Bennett 1995; Hudak 1998). The flush bag is attached to the arterial line via tubing and placed under pressure by utilizing a sleeve which is inflated to 300 mmHg (greater than arterial pressure). This ensures a continuous flush of 3–5 ml/hr (Smith 2000).

Transducers enable the pressure readings from the invasive monitoring of a patient to be displayed on a screen. To ensure accuracy several steps must be taken.

1. The transducer set must be primed before connection to the patient and all air bubbles removed from the system.
2. The transducer must be positioned level with the right atrium and its height altered when patient position changed (Pearson 2002). The same reference point should always be used to ensure meaningful comparison.
3. The use of three-way taps should be limited.
4. Calibration of the transducer to atmospheric pressure should occur prior to use. It is best practice for this also to be complete at each shift handover, encouraging the nurse to check the position of the transducer, promoting accurate blood pressure measurement.

The arterial waveform should have sharp and steady upstrokes caused by steadily increasing pressure as blood is ejected from the left ventricle (Coad 1996). At the end of ventricular contraction systole is reached, represented by the brief peak on the trace. As aortic pressure falls, the aortic valve closes, causing a brief surge in pressure known as the dicrotic notch. Pressure then falls steadily until diastole is reached.

Complications of arterial lines include exsanguination, ischaemia distal to the cannula and tissue necrosis, air embolus and thrombus (Jevon and Ewans 2007). The nurse caring for a child with an arterial line must be vigilant and ensure that the limb is checked at least hourly for signs of reduced perfusion, movement or loss of sensation. Best practice would be for the limb to be exposed for continual observation but this may not always be practical, for example if there is a femoral line in situ. Infection risks with arterial lines tend to be higher as the line is accessed more frequently for blood gas analysis and laboratory investigations (Gwinnutt 2006). On removal of the line, direct pressure should be applied to the insertion point until bleeding stops.

Blood gases

Blood gas analysis is facilitated by the insertion of an arterial line allowing for withdrawal of arterial blood for measurement. Blood gas analysis may be required to allow evaluation of interventions made (such as commencement of non-invasive ventilation), to explain sudden or unexpected deterioration, to manage fluid and electrolyte balance or as a baseline to facilitate postoperative management in a child undergoing major surgery. Before reviewing the basics of blood gas analysis, we must analyse some of the key words used to describe components of blood gases.

An acid is defined as any substance that is capable of providing hydrogen ions (H^+) when it is in a solution (Driscoll *et al.* 1997). Examples of acids found within the body include hydrochloric acid, lactic acid and pyruvic acid.

The opposite of an acid is a base. This is defined as any substance that accepts hydrogen ions when in a solution. Examples of bases produced by the body include bicarbonate, phosphate and ammonia.

An alkali is a substance that can donate hydroxide ions (OH^-). It can also accept hydrogen ions.

pH is a term used to describe the acidity or alkalinity of a solution. The pH scale was developed to express the concentration of hydrogen ions in an easier way. The normal pH of an arterial blood sample is 7.35–7.45 which is equivalent to a hydrogen concentration of 44–36 nmol/l. A pH less than 7.35 is known as an acidosis. A pH greater than 7.45 is known as an alkalosis. 6.8–7.8 is the pH range usually considered compatible with life (Driscoll *et al.* 1997). A normal intracellular pH is required for the functioning of many cellular enzymes that exist in the body. The body has many mechanisms to maintain normal pH and many buffers exist to protect against pH changes.

Within the body, buffers are present which are responsible for regulating the amount of free hydrogen ions available to cause a significant change in pH before they are eliminated from the body. Buffers act to uptake the free hydrogen ions within the bloodstream and the cells of the body. Alternately they can also work to release hydrogen ions when confronted with a strong base, the aim being to maintain a normal pH at all times. Haemoglobin represents an important protein buffer and is effective at both donating and accepting hydrogen ions. Extracellular buffers including plasma proteins and the carbonic acid–bicarbonate system are also key to the body's buffering system.

Proteins act like sponges and soak up hydrogen ions, transporting them to their place of elimination. In the majority of cases this will be the kidneys. In contrast, the carbonic acid–bicarbonate system acts by allowing the extra hydrogen ions to react with bicarbonate to produce carbon dioxide and water:

$$HCO_3 + H^+ \leftrightarrow H_2CO_3 \leftrightarrow CO_2 + H_2O$$

Bicarbonate Ion   Hydrogen ion   Carbonic acid   Carbon dioxide   Water

When analysing blood gas results, consideration to compensatory mechanisms in place within the body's natural ability will be present. For example short-term control of blood pH is exerted via the respiratory system. The respiratory centre is driven by the pH of cerebrospinal fluid (CSF). A drop in CSF pH will be detected and cause an increase in respiratory rate and depth to reduced the amount of CO_2 within the bloodstream. This contributes to a rise in blood pH.

Longer-term control of acid–base balance is exerted by the production of bicarbonate in the kidney and the excretion of acid. An acidic pH causes increased secretion of hydrogen ions which displaces another cation, usually sodium. The cation then combines with bicarbonate to form sodium bicarbonate which is then absorbed into the bloodstream, leading to an increase in pH.

Before analysing abnormalities one must understand the normal range for blood gas values in humans (Table 3.2).

Now that normal ranges are present, representation of common disturbances within blood pH and the compensatory mechanisms in place to correct this are given in Table 3.3.

When analysing a blood gas the first thing to check is the pH. Consider whether it is within normal range. If not, is it acidotic or alkalotic? pH <7.35 is acidotic, while pH >7.45 is considered alkalotic. Next review CO_2 – it is high, low or normal? Deviations from the norm with CO_2 may be suggestive of respiratory insufficiency and interventions may

Table 3.2 Blood gas normal values.

Item	Normal range
pH	7.35–7.34
PCO_2	4.5–6.0 kPa
PO_2	10–12 kPa
HCO_3 (actual bicarbonate)	22–26 mmol/l
Base excess	−2–+2 mmol/l

Table 3.3 Mechanisms in place to correct common disturbances within blood pH.

Acid base disorder	pH	Primary disturbance	Compensatory response
Respiratory acidosis	↓	↑$PaCO_2$	↑HCO_3^- ↑(positive) base excess
Respiratory alkalosis	↑	↓$PaCO_2$	↓HCO_3^- ↓(negative) base excess
Metabolic acidosis	↓	↓HCO_3^- ↓(negative) base excess	↓$PaCO_2$
Metabolic alkalosis	↑	↑HCO_3^- ↑(positive) base excess	↑$PaCO_2$

be required to support this. An increase in CO_2 will lead to a decrease in pH (respiratory acidosis). A decrease in CO_2 will lead to an increase in pH (respiratory alkalosis).

PO_2 should be analysed with blood gas results in conjunction with oxygen requirements and oxygen saturations. The nurse should ensure that saturations are maintained greater than 95% for all patients (unless clinical condition dictates otherwise, for example in certain respiratory or cardiac disorders).

Next consider the bicarbonate. A low bicarbonate and a negative base deficit indicate a metabolic acidosis, whereas a high bicarbonate and positive base are suggestive of a metabolic alkalosis. Compensatory mechanisms may be seen on blood gas analysis, with metabolic disturbances compensated by acute changes in respiratory drive and chronically by renal responses. The actions taken in response to blood gas analysis require a team approach and monitoring of interventions is required. Repeat blood gas analysis may be required after interventions are complete. Blood gas results should be documented in the patient's medical notes (or in a designated place on the observation chart).

Central venous catheters and central venous pressure monitoring

Central venous catheters are commonly placed in children within the high dependency setting. In the UK, approximately 200,000 central venous catheters are inserted each year (National Institute for Clinical Excellence 2002). Indications for central venous catheters include:

- fluid resuscitation
- drug and fluid administration
- parenteral feeding
- measurement of central venous pressure
- poor venous access.

Common sites for insertion include:

- internal jugular vein
- femoral vein
- umbilical vein (neonates)
- subclavian vein (less common).

Risks for children undergoing central line insertion include:

- haemorrhage
- infection
- embolization
- arrhythmias
- pneumothorax.

An experienced member of staff should be present at line insertion as sedation will be required and complications with airway maintenance may occur. The minimum monitoring required is pulse oximetry.

It is recommended that central venous catheters are inserted under ultrasound guidance and this equipment should be available for the use of those involved in this process. Central venous catheters can be single, double, triple or quadruple lumened. Following insertion of these catheters, they should be managed by experienced staff following strict infection control procedures, as microorganisms that colonize catheter hubs and the skin adjacent to the site are the source of most catheter-related bloodstream infections (Department of Health 2001). There are several factors to consider when caring for a patient with a central venous catheter:

- Dress the site with a transparent dressing to allow the site to be frequently visually checked for leakage, redness or swelling. A child with a central venous catheter should also have their temperature recorded at least once daily.
- Ensure any drugs being infused through the line are clearly labelled to minimize risk of bolus infusions.
- Check patency of the lines (at least once per shift) and ensure the line is clamped with a secure connector at the end. If using Bionectors/Smartsites™, ensure documentation of the date that they were connected to the line, to promote timely changes.
- Assess the need for the line at each ward round. Central venous catheters can contribute to morbidity and mortality for seriously ill patients and therefore the catheter should be removed when it is no longer required (Clemence *et al.* 1995; O'Leary and Bihari 1998).

Central venous catheters allow monitoring of central venous pressure (CVP) within the high dependency unit. CVP can be useful in the assessment of cardiac function, circulating blood volume, vascular tone and the patient's response to treatment (Chait *et al.* 1999; Druding 2000; Woodrow 2000). It is important to note that CVP can be affected by a number of factors and should therefore be used in conjunction with other measurements such as heart rate, pulse volume and urine output. An isolated CVP reading can be misleading: it is common practice to record CVP measurements hourly on the observation chart and achieve a trend in readings that may demonstrate a response to treatment (such as fluid challenges, inotropic drugs, etc.) and/or disease progression (Woodrow 2002).

CVP measurement is achieved using a transducer identical to that used for arterial blood pressure monitoring. Double transducer sets can be found in the practice areas which allow the operator to use a single flush bag for both the CVP and arterial transducer sets. The pressure bag should be inflated to 300 mmHg (as with the arterial bag) and the patient monitor zeroed following the same process. Zero point should be the right atrium (therefore the patient can be nursed in the same position to achieve an arterial and CVP reading).

The CVP waveform reflects changes in right atrial pressure during the cardiac cycle. The normal CVP trace has three waves: A, C and V.

- A wave – represents atrial contraction;
- C wave – caused by ventricular contraction against a closed tricuspid valve;
- V wave – atrial filling (Hughes and Tariq 2004).

Texts vary as to what is accorded a normal CVP measurement but its range is approximately 5–12 mmHg (Woodrow 2002; Laight *et al.* 2005).

Nutrition/intravenous therapy

Each child admitted to the high dependency unit will require an individualized assessment with regard to the need for intravenous fluids. Nutrition is essential in children for activity, growth and maintenance tissue repair and this becomes even more important in children who are sick. Ideally, oral intake should be maintained and a balanced diet offered. If this is not easily achieved, consider placing a nasogastric tube and offer enteral feeding via this route. The expertise of a paediatric dietician will be necessary. In some cases, for example after surgery, in children experiencing respiratory distress or those with continued abdominal and bowel dysfunction, the establishment or maintenance of oral/enteral feeding may not be possible. In this instance, intravenous fluids should be commenced.

The content and distribution of water in the human body also changes with age. The water in body tissues is contained within compartments (Willock and Jewkes 2000). Intracellular fluid is water contained within cells. Extracellular fluid is water outside of the cells. Extracellular fluid is further divided into:

- intravascular fluid (plasma)
- interstitial fluid (surrounding tissue cells)
- transcellular fluid (i.e. CSF, pleural, peritoneal fluid).

The movement of fluid between the vascular space and the tissues depends on a variety of pressures, namely osmotic, oncotic and hydrostatic pressures and changes in capillary permeability. Many clinical conditions will cause variations in the movement of fluid between the vascular space and the tissues. The extent of this will need to be assessed in the clinical area using skills of observation, palpation, percussion and auscultation.

Monitoring fluid balance is an important nursing role. Children should have an accurate fluid balance chart detailing input and output on an hourly basis. The total fluid balance should be recorded each hour. Calculating the amount of fluid a patient needs can be difficult, particularly in those who are sick and may require supplemental fluid boluses to maintain normal cardiovascular function. Table 3.4 is a guide to the fluid requirements of children within the high dependency unit.

One of the most common reasons for admission to hospital is dehydration secondary to diarrhoea and vomiting. An adjunct to your assessment of fluid requirement will be to establish the degree of dehydration:

- Mild (<5% loss of bodyweight) – few clinical signs, perhaps dry tongue, flat fontanelle.

Table 3.4 Fluid requirement based on weight.

Child's weight	Kilogram body weight formula
Newborn – up to 72 hrs after birth	60–100 ml/kg
Up to 10 kg	100 ml/kg (may be increased to 150 ml/kg on clinician assessment)
11–20 kg	1000 ml for 1st 10 kg + 50 ml/kg for each kg over 10 kg
21–30 kg	1500 ml for the first 20 kg + 20 ml/kg for each kg over 20 kg (some units may choose to use 25 ml/kg over 20 kg)

- Moderate (5–10% loss of body weight) – obvious clinical signs of loss of interstitial fluid; sunken fontanelle, tachycardia, dry tongue.
- Severe (10–15% loss of body weight) – seriously ill; weak fast pulse, low blood pressure, poor urine output.

Children who are solely dependent on intravenous fluid will need supplementation of electrolytes such as sodium, potassium, calcium and phosphate. Serum blood levels should be checked regularly, at least once in a 24-hour period, as this will help to guide the fluid regime over the next 12–24 hours (Gosling 1999). Patients who have received intravenous fluids for several days with no progression towards oral/enteral feeding should be considered for alternative nutrition, for example intravenous total parental nutrition (TPN). A paediatric dietician should be routinely involved in the care of all patients within the high dependency unit.

Serum electrolytes for those children requiring supplementation of nutrition in the form of intravenous fluids or total parental nutrition should be analysed at least every 24 hours. Table 3.5 is a summary of commonly analysed electrolytes and their normal ranges.

Electrocardiograms

ECG monitoring provides a continuous picture of the heart's electrical activity, which includes the heart rate and rhythm. A child's heart rate varies dependent not only on age, but also the level of activity in which they are participating (Table 3.6).

The contraction of any muscle is associated with electrical changes called depolarization, and these changes can be detected by electrodes attached to the surface of the body. Correct electrode placement is vital to obtain accurate information. Most high dependency settings use a

Table 3.5 Commonly analysed electrolytes and their normal ranges. Adapted from Avidan *et al.* (2008) and Blann (2007).

Electrolyte	Normal range	Function
Sodium (Na⁺)	133–148 mmol/l	Primary electrolyte in blood. Major contributor to the osmolarity of blood
Potassium (K⁺)	3.3–5.6 mmol/l	Intracellular ion. Plays key role in membrane activity
Calcium (Ca⁺⁺)	2.19–2.51 mmol/l	Variety of crucial roles in cell signalling, neural function, muscle contraction and blood coagulation. 98% located in bone
Magnesium (Mg⁺)	0.65–0.95 mmol/l	Predominantly intracellular ion with roles such as cofactor for various enzymes, muscle contractility and neuronal transmission

Table 3.6 Normal heart rates in children.

Age	Awake HR (per min)	Sleeping HR (per minute)
Neonate	100–180	80–160
Infant (6 month)	100–160	75–160
Toddler	80–110	60–90
Preschool	70–110	60–90
School-age child	65–110	60–90
Adolescent	60–90	50–90

three-wire monitoring system. Suggested ECG electrode placement is red (right shoulder), yellow (left shoulder) and green (left lower thorax or hip region) (Jacobson 2000). The ECG functions in four stages:

1. The sinus node fires and the electrical impulse spread across the atria. This results in artial contraction (P wave).
2. On arriving at the AV junction the impulse is delayed, allowing the atria time to contract and eject blood into the ventricles.
3. The impulse is then conducted down to the ventricles through the bundle of His, right and left bundle branches and Purkinje fibres causing ventricular depolarization and contraction (QRS complex).
4. The ventricles then repolarize (T wave) (Jevon and Ewens 2007).

Arrhythmias are deviations from the normal (sinus) rhythm of the heart. Arrhythmias in children with no underlying cardiac disease are rare but may be seen during critical illness. Common arrhythmias include bradyarrhythmias and tachyarrhythmias. Arrhythmias will be examined more closely in Chapter 5.

ECG electrodes should be changed daily as the contact gel can dry out and occasionally contact burns can be noted on a child's skin. If the monitor is displaying an abnormal or absent rate and rhythm you should first assess the patient, ensuring that a pulse is present. Once clinical assessment has established that the patient has a regular rate and rhythm, check electrode placement, ensure that the wires are attached correctly and that monitoring is occurring through lead 2 (on the monitoring device). This will usually result in an ECG trace being achieved.

Pulse oximetry

Pulse oximetry is widely used within healthcare settings with the main aim being to detect hypoxaemia before it can be detected by sight or before obvious symptoms are displayed. The pulse oximeter provides continuous, non-invasive monitoring of the oxygen saturation in haemoglobin in arterial blood. Pulse oximetry only measures the extent to which haemoglobin is saturated with oxygen and does not provide information on oxygen delivery to the tissues or ventilatory function (Higgins 2005).

The pulse oximeter consists of two light-emitting diodes (one infrared and one red) on one side of the probe. These transmit red and infrared light across the tissue bed (usually finger or toe), to a photo detector on the other side of the probe (Welch 2005). The ratio of absorption is relative to the concentration of oxygenated haemoglobin to deoxygenated haemoglobin (Chandler 2000). The more oxygenated the blood, the more red light passes through. By calculating the ratios of red to infrared light over time, oxygen saturation is calculated (Giuliano 2006).

The normal range for children (other than those with a known cardiac aetiology or chronic lung disease) is >95% (Fox 2002; Booker 2004). There are many different probe types used in practice. Common sites in children include:

- finger or toe (using self-adhesive probe or finger probe)
- the ear lobe (using clip probe)
- across the palm of the hand (in smaller children)
- across the foot (in smaller children).

It is important that the area utilized should be cleaned and nail varnish removed to ensure accuracy of readings (Whaley and Wong 1999).

The infrared light should shine down through the skin, and on the opposite side the photo detector should be able to pick up a reading. The pulse oximeter screen should display a wave with a numerical reading at the end. If there is no wave form, the reading will not be accurate (this may be seen when there is poor tissue perfusion at the site used for measurement).

Other causes of inaccuracies with readings include:

- carbon monoxide poisoning whereby falsely high readings may be obtained;
- venous pulsation if the probe is secured too tightly or a blood pressure cuff is inflated above the probe site, leading to a falsely low reading;
- factors that affect light absorption such as skin pigmentation, dried blood and intravenous dyes;
- movement by the patient such as shivering can lead to a falsely low reading or a inaccurate reading due to a poor trace;
- oxygen saturations less than 70% are unable to be accurately measured through pulse oximetry (Schnapp and Cohen 1990).

Probe sites should be changed frequently in practice as it has been documented that children may experience pressure sores and even superficial burns when probes have been left in situ for long periods. Best practice is to change them 4–6 hourly. Always note the use of supplementary oxygen when recording pulse oximetry and ensure an accurate trace is obtained when taking readings. Be aware of the effect that movement can have, particularly when dealing with children, and ensure that you observe skin colour and pallor alongside pulse oximeter readings. Observational assessment provides information on the accuracy of the pulse oximetry reading and must be considered when interpreting oxygen saturation levels.

Oxygen administration

Oxygen is commonly used for children with respiratory disease. It is important that the correct method of administration is chosen, for both the age and the condition of the child. The child will also need monitoring with pulse oximetry and regular respiratory assessment if they are receiving oxygen. You should also record the amount of oxygen being delivered to the child either in litres per minute or as a concentration – FiO_2. Oxygen should be regarded as a drug and should therefore be prescribed on the drug prescription chart (BMJ Publishing 2006).

Factors to take into consideration when choosing oxygen delivery method:

- age of child
- clinical condition of child
- percentage/flow rate of oxygen prescribed
- compliance of child.

There are some complications that can occur when administering oxygen to children and these need to be taken into consideration. They are usually related to suboptimal delivery and monitoring techniques (Pease 2006). It is important to ensure that monitoring is reliable and accurate as this is being used as a method to assess the effectiveness of the oxygen therapy. Prolonged use of dry oxygen at high flow rates can cause drying of the mucous membranes which can lead to discomfort for the child. Oxygen toxicity can also be a problem and is caused when high levels of oxygen are delivered unnecessarily. The oxygen flow or concentration should be titrated to achieve a normal oxygen saturation of 95%. Care must also be taken when administering oxygen to children who may normally have a lower oxygen saturation level, such as children with chronic airway disease or cardiac disease. It is important to establish what a normal saturation level is for these children and titrate the oxygen to achieve this. Artificially increasing the oxygen saturation level can be very dangerous for such children.

Nasal cannulae

Nasal cannulae are useful for infants who are obligatory nose breathers or for older children when a high percentage or fast flow of oxygen is required. Cannulae can deliver up to 2 litres per minute. They allow the child to feed and still receive oxygen. Humidification is not necessary as the gas is entering via the nasal passages where it is warmed and moistened. Ill-fitting cannulae can obstruct the nostrils so care needs to be taken that the correct size is chosen. They should occupy less than half the space in the nasal passage. Care also needs to be taken to ensure that the nostrils and the face do not become sore from the cannula. There is limited oxygen delivery available with this method, with the child receiving about 28% FiO_2 (Field 2005) when 2 litres per minute is delivered through the device.

Head box

Head boxes are very useful for delivering high concentrations of oxygen to infants. They can reliably deliver oxygen concentrations of up to 90%. They also provide high humidity as the oxygen must be humidified and warmed prior to it entering the head box. This is important as the temperature of the infant can be compromised if the oxygen is not warmed. The oxygen concentration in the head box can be monitored, so allowing accurate recording of how much oxygen the infant requires. An oxygen analyser should be placed inside the head box to provide accurate measurement of the concentration of oxygen delivered to the child. It is very important that the opening of the head box where the infant is positioned is not obstructed in any way. Obstruction can lead to a build-up of exhaled carbon dioxide in the box and thus a decrease in oxygen concentration. The disadvantages of a head box are that the infant can be difficult to observe and it can create a barrier between infant and parents. The infant also needs to lie relatively still within the box. The infant will need to be removed for oral feeding and care, so it can be difficult to maintain a consistent level of oxygenation.

Simple face mask

This device delivers approximately 35–60% FiO_2 with a flow rate between 6 and 12 litres per minute (a minimum flow of 6 litres per minute should be maintained to prevent rebreathing of exhaled carbon dioxide). By utilizing elephant tubing, water and a heater, humidification can be achieved via this device. The insertion of an oxygen flow meter can also control the percentage of oxygen delivered and assist the practitioner in assessing the amount of oxygen required for the child to maintain normal or improved oxygen saturations. The mask should be the correct size to ensure a good fit, enabling optimum oxygen delivery. The mask comes in two sizes, paediatric and adult, and is therefore not appropriate for infants and smaller children. Rebreathing of CO_2 does occur with this device and the amount of oxygen received by the child is dependent on their respiratory effort, particularly the rate and tidal volume. Indications for this device may be simple postoperative recovery and short-term use.

Non-rebreathe masks with reservoir bags

This is a face mask with a reservoir bag attached. There are either one or two valves over the exhalation ports on the mask, allowing approximately 95–100% FiO_2 to be delivered. To achieve this the reservoir bag is connected to an oxygen supply, usually delivered at 15 litres per minute, which causes it to inflate and fill. The reservoir has a valve preventing exhaled air from entering and blocking entrainment of gas from the atmosphere on inspiration, ensuring that only supplemental oxygen contained within the reservoir bag is inhaled by the patient. Exhaled gas is directed out from the side ports on the mask. Oxygen delivered cannot be humidified and therefore drying out of the oral/nasal pharynx will occur. However, this device should be used as a short-term adjunct to oxygen delivery and the child must have continuous respiratory assessment if requiring this level of supplemental oxygen. Medical staff must be alerted to the amount of FiO_2 delivered to maintain normal oxygen saturations. It may be necessary for further respiratory support to be instigated (such as non-invasive ventilation).

Humidification

Humidification is important in the delivery of oxygen, primarily because it prevents the mucous membranes from drying out. Any oxygen that is going to be delivered for longer than 6 hours should be humidified. There are various methods by which the oxygen can be humidified. Different connectors are available from manufacturers that enable the oxygen delivery system to be connected to a disposable water bottle. The nasal cannulae connection is a simple snap-off valve that enables the cannulae to be connected directly to the water bottle. There are also adaptors available that allow the delivery of oxygen as a percentage. These are usually used with elephant tubing. It is important to follow the manufacturer's instructions and change the water delivery bottles at regular intervals. This is to prevent infection. The normal period of use is 24 hours. Most humidification systems also allow the oxygen to be warmed. This is important if the child is going to receive the oxygen for a prolonged period of time.

Temperature

Children within the high dependency unit requiring frequent monitoring of their temperature and this should be performed 4 hourly as a minimum (Andrews and Nolan 2006). Normal body temperature is usually between 36 °C and 37.5 °C (Trim 2005). The body's core temperature is usually the highest, while the skin is the coolest.

There are many electronic devices available for measuring body temperature in children. These devices are considered safe and are fast to use (Tortora and Grabowski 1996). The most commonly used within the high dependency unit are tympanic thermometers and oral/axilla thermometers.

Tympanic thermometers

The tympanic membrane shares the same carotid blood supply as the hypothalamus, hence the measurement of temperature here should reflect the core temperature (Woodrow 2000). The tympanic thermometer is designed for intermittent use, giving a one-off digital reading.

Readings from a tympanic thermometer that seem low may be due to ineffective use of the device. Problems often occur when trying to use it on a smaller child when achieving a snug fit into the ear canal is not possible. Alternative measuring devices must be considered for the younger age group.

Oral/axilla thermometers

These routes are frequently used in practice for measuring a child's temperature. If choosing the oral route, place the probe under the tongue of the child, asking them to close their mouth firmly. The probe should be placed under the sublingual pocket of tissue at the base of the tongue, not the area at the front as this may lead to a lower reading. If the child is unable to follow commands it may be necessary to use the axilla for temperature measurement. Select axilla measurement on the device. Place the probe in the centre of the armpit with the patient's arm positioned firmly against the side of the chest.

There are several problems that can occur when measuring temperatures in children. When using the oral route, a falsely low reading may be obtained if the probe is positioned incorrectly. It can be difficult to explain to a child the position the probe should be maintained and children often move the probe around within their mouth. The axilla route can also be difficult to obtain an accurate measurement as the site is not close to a major blood vessel and the surface temperature of the skin can be affected by the environment (Woollens 1996). Measurement of temperature using a tympanic device is inappropriate for a smaller child due to the inability to ensure a seal around the ear canal, hence the nurse must use clinical judgement to determine the most appropriate measurement tool for the child. Document the site at which the temperature was recorded and ensure this method and route is used for further measurement so that a trend can be analysed.

Analysis of temperature via the rectal route is a method almost obsolete within paediatric nursing. It is occasionally used within paediatric resuscitations, particularly submersion events when active rewarming is performed under controlled conditions and temperature measurement is vital.

Wound management

Children admitted to the high dependency unit may have either surgical or traumatic wounds that will need to be cared for. It is important to consider the anatomy and physiology of the skin as this will enable optimal wound healing to take place through correct wound care. The skin is composed of two major layers of tissue:

- the outer epidermis which provides protection, and prevents micro-organisms from entering the body;
- the inner dermis, which is composed of blood vessels and accessory structures (hair, nails, sweat glands and sebaceous glands), and collagen fibres and elastin which give the skin its strength and flexibility.

The functions of the skin are:

- Protection of underlying organs and tissues from mechanical damage.
- Excretion of excess salts, water and urea from the body.
- Temperature regulation.
- Maintenance of body shape. The elasticity of skin restores the shape when joints are used during movement.
- Protection against excessive loss of water from the body by evaporation.
- Protection against entry of harmful organisms.
- Storage of nutrients.
- Detection of stimuli such as temperature, pain and touch and the relay of this information to the nervous system.

Wound healing can happen in two ways: by primary intention or by secondary intention. In primary intention wound healing, the wound edges are opposed as soon as possible, there is no tissue loss and healing is rapid. The granulated tissue is not visible and scar formation is minimal. In secondary intention wound healing, granulation occurs where damage to the epithelium has been sustained.

Wound healing occurs in three stages:

1. The inflammatory stage: response (24–48 hrs) – yellow slough on the wound surface and some redness around the wound margins.
2. The granulation or proliferation stage – granulation tissue begins to form along with epithelialization until the wound bed is filled. There is a red wound surface which bleeds easily if the fragile new capillary bed is disturbed.
3. The maturation stage – the wound continues to strengthen for 12 months or more as the scar tissue is rearranged and strengthened.

Wound assessment needs to be undertaken both on admission and at regular intervals. Any changes noted to the wound including

Table 3.7 Use of appropriate wound dressings for wound type.

Wound type	Dressing
Dry necrotic wounds	Hydrocolloids and hydrogels
Sough covered wounds	Hydrocolloids and hydrogels
Clean exuding wounds (granulating)	Hydrocolloids, foams, alginates
Clean, dry low exudate wounds (epithelializing)	Absorbent perforated plastic film-faced dressing Vapour-permeable adhesive film dressings
Clean medium to high exudate wounds (epithelializing)	Knitted varicose primary dressing Paraffin gauze

increased redness, pain, swelling or exudate should lead to the wound being reassessed. Wound assessment consists of the following components:

- The position and size of the wound, and the wound etiology
- The tissue type (e.g. sloughy, necrotic, granulating, or epithelializing)
- The amount of exudate
- The presence or absence of infection
- The presence or absence of pain
- The possibility of a sinus.

Once the wound has been assessed then an appropriate dressing needs to be chosen. Table 3.7 identifies appropriate wound dressings for different wound types.

In order for wound healing to be successful the following conditions need to be met for the wound:

1. Moist
2. Free from exudates
3. Free from dead tissue
4. Free from effects of trauma
5. Warm
6. Protected
7. Acidic.

Choice of dressing is therefore crucial when managing wounds. Other factors that need to be considered when managing children's wounds are procedural pain management during the dressing changes and the suitability of the dressing for the child's age and range of movement.

> ## Case study: 1-year-old with diarrhoea and vomiting
>
> A 1-year-old child is brought into the Emergency Department with a 2-day history of diarrhoea and vomiting. The child's mother reports that he has not had oral intake for 12 hours and that he is irritable and has no energy this morning. His mother says the nappy that was put onto the child before he went to bed was still dry when she woke him up.

Management

Let's consider a structured approach to the assessment of this child. An AVPU and ABC approach should be initially followed.

AVPU
In this instance the child is drowsy (AVPU = V).

Airway and breathing

- Is the child's airway patent? Yes.
- Is he making vocal sounds? Yes.
- Is there anything abnormal around the nose and mouth? No.
- If the airway is patent, is the child spontaneously breathing? Yes.
- Count the respiratory rate and observe the effort of breathing.
- Is the respiratory rate within normal parameters? No.
- Is the child using any accessory muscles to assist respiratory effort? No.
- Document respiratory rate and signs of increased effort such as nasal flaring, use of accessory muscles and tracheal tug.
- Having established that the child is breathing, additional monitoring may be required. Auscultate the child's chest.
- Are there breath sounds throughout? Yes.
- Are any additional noises present? No.
- Palpate the child's chest, comparing left and right side. Are any abnormalities detected? No.
- Percussion of the child's chest may be performed but this is not often well tolerated in the younger age group. In this instance the child has a respiratory rate of 55/minute.
- Place a pulse oximetry probe on to the child's finger or toe (an accurate reading may be difficult to achieve if the child has cool

peripheries). In this instance the oxygen saturation is 94% so a simple paediatric size face mask is applied and the saturation improves to 99%.

Circulation

- Look at the child's colour – is the child pink? Mottled? Cyanosed? The child has cool mottled peripheries.
- Check central and peripheral capillary refill. Remember to hold the limb used for peripheral refill above the level of the heart and press for a 5s period. Compare central refill time. Common site used for this is the child's trunk. Is circulation restored within <2s? No, in this instance the capillary refill time is 5 seconds.
- What is the child's heart rate and rhythm? In this instance the heart rate is 175/minute and regular on palpation.
- Feel both central and peripheral pulses. How do they compare? Thready at the brachial site, slightly fuller volume at the femoral site.
- Place ECG electrodes to aid assessment of rate and rhythm. Auscultate the heart. Are they any additional sounds other than S1 and S2? In this instance the ECG demonstrates a sinus tachycardia and the heart sounds are regular with no additional noises.

Intravenous access is now required. Cardiovascular compromise is evident, therefore intravenous access should be immediately sought with two large peripheral cannulae being the gold standard within this situation. If intravenous access is unsuccessful an intraosseous cannula should be placed without delay. Once access is sought, blood samples should be sent. In particular blood sugar, U&Es and a blood gas should be obtained. Due to cardiovascular instability a fluid bolus should be administered. Standard practice is to administer a 20ml/kg bolus of 0.9% saline.

After the 20ml/kg bolus is administered, assessment must be revisited. Start from A (airway) and work through the systems, following the same approach. It is vital that airway and breathing are maintained otherwise circulation will fail regardless of the clinician's effort. Utilize the team around you and the monitoring devices you have to aid clinical observation. Is the airway patent? Child still breathing? Adequate respiratory effort? Is the child pink? What is the heart rate? Any change since the fluid bolus? Capillary refill time? Does the child have warm hands and feet? Is the child more responsive? It is likely that a reduction in heart rate may be witnessed but a second fluid bolus of 20ml/kg saline may be required.

In this instance the blood sugar is 2.4mmol. Hypoglycaemia is common in sick infants and should be treated promptly with 5ml/kg of 10% dextrose solution intravenous. A subsequent test demonstrates improvement to 6.1 mmol.

The child's temperature could also be taken here. The child will have to be exposed for assessment and may require additional warming devices to maintain normothermia.

Blood gas analysis will be instant. On this occasion the blood gas result is:

pH	7.27
pCO_2	3.5
pO_2	11.5
HCO_3	18.3
BE	−6

This blood gas shows an acidosis (pH < 7.35). Next look at the respiratory component of the gas. This shows a lower than normal CO_2 which would normally lead to an alkalosis if only the respiratory component were affected; however, analyse the metabolic component of the gas. We can see a negative base excess and low bicarbonate (contributing to the acidotic pH). This blood gas demonstrates the compensatory mechanisms contributing to the maintenance of a normal pH within the human body. Having recognized that the blood pH has changed, the respiratory centre has increased the child's respiratory rate, contributing to a reduced pCO_2. As carbon dioxide is an acid, expulsion of this will artificially increase the blood pH until the metabolic component is corrected. As the child receives supplemental fluid boluses, the metabolic acidosis will begin to correct and the child's respiratory rate should reduce back to within normal parameters to maintain normal pCO_2 limits.

Common findings in a child whom has reduced oral intake for a period of time is a delayed capillary refill time, increased heart rate and difference in pulse volumes when comparing peripheral and central (central pulse volume is normally maintained until severe dehydration occurs and cardiovascular collapse is present). Peripheral pulse volume is weak and thready. The diagnosis is compensated hypovolaemic shock. Following the initial fluid resuscitation the child will need to be adequately rehydrated over a period of 24–48 hours. For this to be achieved the child will need to be admitted to hospital. As the child's neurological status was affected and several fluid boluses have been administered, the child is likely to be admitted to the high dependency unit for close observation. Standard practice is that a child receiving 40–60 ml/kg of fluid should be monitored within a HDU/PICU as additional respiratory and circulatory support may be necessary. Clinical assessment is vital to ensure accurate management of this child and monitoring tools to assist this include ECG, pulse oximetry, blood pressure reading and blood gas analysis.

Conclusion

Within the high dependency unit it will be necessary to utilize various monitoring devices and interventions to support the clinical assessment and management of a child's condition. Never underestimate the benefit of actual 'hands on' assessment, that is clinical inspection, auscultation, percussion and palpation as described throughout this book. Monitoring devices are simply adjuncts to support this assessment. Earlier subtle signs will have been demonstrated, for example lethargy and irritability, that will not be picked up by monitoring devices alone. A practitioner working within a high dependency unit requires the skills and knowledge to ensure correct utilization and evaluation of the monitoring devices available. Recognition of the limitations of monitoring devices has been discussed within this chapter and the high dependency practitioner may need to consider alternative methods to ensure accurate measurement of clinical parameters.

Learning activities

- Consider the therapeutic interventions that you carry out in the clinical area where you work and the nursing care required. Reflect upon whether the interventions are performed appropriately.
- Reflect upon the care you have provided for a child requiring multiple interventions. How did you ensure the child was allowed to rest adequately and did not become too distressed?
- Reflect upon the explanations that you give to families and children when carrying out therapeutic interventions. Do they understand the need for the intervention?

References and further reading

Andrews F, Nolan J (2006) Critical care in the emergency department: monitoring the critically ill patient. *Emergency Medicine Journal* **23**: 561–564.

Avidan M, Barnett KM, Hill LL, Hopley L, Jones N, Van Schalkwyk JM (2008) *Intensive Care: an illustrated colour text*. Elsevier, London.

Blann A (2007) Routine Blood Results Explained: a guide for nurses and allied health professinals, 2nd Edition. M&K Update Ltd, Keswick, Cumbria.

BMJ Publishing Group (2006) *British National Formulary for Children*. www.bnfc.org. BMJ Publishing Group/RPS Publishing/RCPCH Publications, London.

Booker R (2004) The effective assessment of acute breathlessness in a patient. *Nursing Times* **100**(24): 61.

British Hypertension Society (2006) *Blood Pressure Measurement*. www.bhsoc. org (accessed 07/05/08).

Campbell B (1997) Arterial waveforms: monitoring changes in configuration. *Heart and Lung* **26**(3): 205–215.

Chait HI, Kuhn MA, Baum VC (1999) Inferior vena caval pressures predict right atrial pressure in pediatric cardiac surgical patients. *Critical Care Medicine* **27**: 219–224.

Chandler T (2000) Oxygen saturation monitoring. *Paediatric Nursing* **12**(8): 37–42.

Clemence M, Walker D, Farr B (1995) Central venous catheter practice: results of a survey. *American Journal of Infection Control* **23**(1): 5–12.

Coad S (1996) Cardiovascular needs. In Viney C (ed.) *Nursing the Critically Ill.* Bailliere Tindall, London: 77–119.

Department of Health (2001) Guidelines for preventing infections associated with the insertion and maintenance of central venous catheters. *Journal of Hospital Infection* **47** (supplement): S47–S67.

Driscoll P, Brown T, Gwinnutt C, Wardle T (1997) *A Simple Guide to Blood Gas Analysis*. BMJ Publishing Group, London.

Druding MC (2000) Integrating haemodynamic monitoring and physical assessment. *Dimensions of Critical Care Nursing* **19**(4): 25–30.

Fox N (2002) Pulse oximetry. *Nursing Times* **98**(40): 65–67.

Gamby A, Bennett J (1995) Feasibility study of the use of non-heparinised 0.9% sodium chloride for transduced arterial and venous lines. *Intensive and Critical Care Nursing* **11**(3): 148–150.

Garretson S (2005) Haemodynamic monitoring: arterial catheters. *Nursing Standard* **19**(31): 55–63.

Giuliano KK (2006) Knowledge of pulse oximetry amongst critical care nurses. *Dimensions of Critical Care Nursing* **25**(1): 44–49.

Gosling P (1999) Fluid balance in the critically ill: the sodium and water audit. *Care of the Critically Ill* **15**(1): 11–18.

Gwinnutt C (2006) *Clinical Anaesthesia*, 2nd Edition. Blackwell Publishing, Oxford.

Higgins D (2005) Pulse oximetry. *Nursing Times* **101**(6): 34.

Hinds CJ, Watson D (1999) ABC of intensive care: circulatory support. *British Medical Journal* **318**: 1749–1752.

Hudak C (1998) Assessment: cardiovascular system. In Hudak C, Gallo B, Benz J (eds) *Critical Care Nursing: a holistic approach*, 5th Edition. J.B. Lippincott Company, Philadelphia: 124–135.

Hughes J, Tariq A (2004) Understanding simple monitoring in paediatric intensive care. *Current Paediatrics* **14**: 459–464.

Jacobson C (2000) Optimum bedside cardiac monitoring. *Progress in Cardiovascular Nursing* **15**(4): 134–137.

Jevon P, Ewens B (2007) *Monitoring the Critically Ill Patient*, 2nd Edition. Blackwell Publishing, Oxford.

Jones DW, Appel LJ, Sheps SG, Rocella EL, Lenfant C (2003) Measuring blood pressure accurately. *JAMA* **289**(8): 1027–1030.

Laight S, Currie M, Davies N (2005) Cardiac care. In Sheppard M, Wright M (eds) *Principles and Practice of High Dependency Nursing*, 2nd Edition. Elsevier, Edinburgh: 123–158.

Lodato RF (1998) Arterial pressure monitoring. In Tobin MJ (ed.) *Principles and Practice of Intensive Care Monitoring*. McGraw-Hill Companies, New York, London: 733–756.

National Institute for Clinical Excellence (2002) NICE guidance on the use of ultrasound locating devices for placing central venous catheters. NICE, London.

O'Brien E, Beevers D, Marshall H (1995) *ABC of Hypertension*. BMJ Books, London.

O'Leary M, Bihari D (1998) Central venous catheters – time for change? *British Medical Journal* **316**: 1918–1919.

Pearson G (2002) *Handbook of Paediatric Intensive Care*. W.B. Saunders, London.

Pease P (2006) Oxygen administration: is practice based on evidence? *Paediatric Nursing* **18**(8) 14–18.

Reeves RA (1995) Does this patient have hypertension? How to measure blood pressure. *JAMA* **273**(5): 1211–1218.

Schnapp LM, Cohen NH (1990) Pulse oximetry: uses and abuses. *Chest* **98**: 1244–1250.

Smith G (2000) Devices for blood pressure measurement. *Professional Nurse* **15**(5): 337–340.

Torrance C, Semple M (1997) Blood pressure measurement. *Nursing Times* **93**(38): suppl. 1–2.

Tortora GJ, Grabowski R (1996) *Principles of Anatomy and Physiology*, 8th Edition. Harper Collins, New York.

Trim J (2005) Monitoring temperature. *Nursing Times* **101**(20): 30–31.

Welch J (2005) Pulse oximeters. *Biomedical Instrumentation and Technology*. March/April: 125–130.

Whaley L, Wong D (1999) *Nursing Care of Infants and Children*, 6th Edition. Mosby, Missouri, MO.

Willock J, Jewkes F (2000) Making sense of fluid balance in children. *Paediatric Nursing* **12**(7): 37–42.

Woodrow P (2000) Arterial blood pressure monitoring. In Moore T, Woodrow P (eds) *High Dependency Nursing Care: observation, intervention and support*. Routledge, London: 301–308.

Woodrow P (2002) Central venous catheters and central venous pressure. *Nursing Standard* **16**(26): 45–51.

Woollens S (1996) Temperature measuring devices. *Professional Nurse* **11**(8): 541–547.

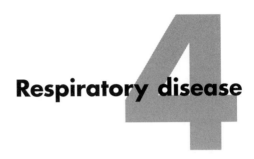

Respiratory disease

Andrea Cockett

Learning outcomes

- To develop an understanding of normal respiratory physiology
- To develop an understanding of how to undertake a respiratory assessment
- To develop an understanding of common interventions used for children with respiratory disease
- To develop an understanding of common respiratory conditions and their management

Introduction

The aim of this chapter is to provide an overview of the common respiratory problems that children may present with in a high dependency setting. Many of the interventions that children require for respiratory disease are similar so these will be covered along with the specific signs, symptoms and interventions required for the most common respiratory problems. At the end of the chapter you should have a good understanding of the common respiratory problems that children present with and the nursing interventions required to care for children with respiratory disease.

Respiratory physiology

In order to provide the nursing interventions required it is necessary to have a good understanding of respiratory anatomy and
physiology.

The respiratory system comprises of:

- the nose
- nasopharynx
- larynx
- bronchi
- the lungs.

The respiratory system is situated in the thorax, and is responsible
for gaseous exchange between the circulatory system and the outside
world. Air is taken in via the upper airways (the nasal cavity, pharynx
and larynx) through the lower airways (trachea, primary bronchi and
bronchial tree) and into the small bronchioles and alveoli within the
lung tissue.

The lungs are divided into lobes. The left lung is composed of the
upper lobe, the lower lobe and the lingula (a small remnant next to the
apex of the heart); the right lung is composed of the upper, the middle
and the lower lobes.

To take a breath in, the external intercostal muscles contract, moving
the ribcage up and out. The diaphragm moves down at the same time,
creating negative pressure within the thorax. The lungs are held to the
thoracic wall by the pleural membranes, and so expand outwards as
well. This creates negative pressure within the lungs, and so air rushes
in through the upper and lower airways.

Expiration is mainly due to the natural elasticity of the lungs,
which tend to collapse if they are not held against the thoracic wall.
This describes the normal mechanism of breathing for an older child.
Infants and younger children have some developmental differences
in their respiratory systems which can affect their clinical
condition.

Infants have large heads with a prominent occiput, which can make
it difficult to position their heads when trying to maintain an open
airway. They have small nostrils and their adenoids and tonsils are
frequently enlarged; this means that any type of mucous blockage or
foreign body inhalation can block the airway. The larynx is short and
narrow and the tongue is large in proportion to the mouth. The nar-
rowest part of the airway is at the cricoid cartilage and the airway itself
is funnel-shaped rather than being cylindrical in shape. The trachea is
short and lung volumes are small in relation to metabolic demand.
Small children also have a small functional residual capacity. Infants

are obligate nose breathers for the first 3 to 6 months of life; they also use their diaphragms to breathe instead of their intercostal muscles. All of these anatomical factors need to be taken into consideration when assessing and caring for infants and young children with respiratory disease.

The primary function of the respiratory system is to facilitate oxygen delivery to the body and allow the elimination of carbon dioxide. The lungs are responsible for exchange of oxygen and carbon dioxide which contributes to the maintenance of acid–base balance. Both gases move between the air and the blood by the process of diffusion. This takes place within the alveoli in the lungs. The alveoli are in direct contact with the pulmonary circulation so allowing the movement of gas from the lungs to the bloodstream. Oxygen binds to the haemoglobin in the red blood cells. When combined with the haemoglobin it becomes oxyhaemoglobin. In order for the haemoglobin to be fully saturated, all four iron atoms that are present in the haem must be combined with oxygen. It is then said to be fully saturated.

Breathing consists of two components:

- Ventilation: the mechanical process of moving air in and out of the lungs, sometimes referred to as the work of breathing;
- Respiration: the exchange of gases within the lungs to supply the tissues and organs with the oxygen they require and to remove carbon dioxide.

Children with respiratory disease can have difficulty with either or both of these processes.

Respiratory assessment

Respiratory assessment may need to be rapid if the condition of the child is poor or the child is distressed.

History

History taking in respiratory assessment can give many vital clues that can aid diagnosis. If the child is stable then taking the history from the parents and child can happen immediately. However, if the child is unable to maintain their own airway or is showing signs of respiratory distress then the history taking will need to be done at a more appropriate time once the child is stabilized.

History taking for respiratory disease has two components: the presenting complaint and the past history.

The presenting complaint

- Was there a preceding illness or was the onset sudden?
- Is there a cough, wheeze or stridor?
- Are there difficulties with feeding?
- Is there associated vomiting?
- Are there symptoms other than respiratory symptoms?

Past history

- Neonatal history – was the child born preterm?
- Has the child had any similar episodes?
- Does the child have a diagnosis of asthma?
- Are the child's immunizations up to date?

Family history

- Any history of asthma, hayfever, eczema?
- Are there any siblings or other family members with similar illnesses?

Social history

- Is the child exposed to tobacco smoke?
- Does the family have any pets?

Medication

- Is the child using any medication?
- Have the parents administered any medication?

Once the history is established you can move on to the physical assessment of the child.

The first and most important area of the assessment is the airway of the child. To check that the airway is patent you need to look for signs of breathing, listen for sounds of breathing and feel for breathing by feeling the chest wall. If these are not present then you need to open the child's airway and call for immediate help. In order to open the airway of an infant you need to tilt the head to a neutral position (sniffing the morning air) and lift the chin. For a child a more pronounced head-tilt chin-lift manouvre is required. Once the airway is secure or the child is able to maintain it for themselves then you need to move on to assess breathing.

Inspection

Respiratory assessment begins with inspection. You need to observe the respiratory rate of the child, counting the number of respirations

Table 4.1 Normal respiratory values in children.

Age	Respirations
<1 years	30–40
1–2 years	25–35
2–5 years	25–30
5–12 years	20–25
>12 years	15–20

over a minute (see Table 4.1). The chest should be inspected to observe the depth of the respiratory movement and also if the movement is symmetrical. Any extra or abnormal movements should be noted. The skin should also be observed for colour. Are the nails, lips and limbs pink or are they dusky or cyanosed? The amount of effort involved in breathing should also be observed. Is the child struggling to breathe? Extra movements that may be noted include head bobbing and intercostal recession. Tracheal tug and nasal flaring may also be present.

The child's level of consciousness should also be observed.

Auscultation

Auscultation is the next step in respiratory assessment. The stethoscope should be placed over the front of the chest to listen to the top two lobes of the lungs. It should then be placed lower on the chest to the sides to listen to the air entry in the lower lobes. The back of the chest should also be listened to. Note should be made of any extra sounds that can be heard. Air should be heard all over the lung fields; if it is not, this shows reduced air entry. This may be just on one side or on both sides. One-sided loss of air entry would indicate obstruction on one side either by swelling, an object or infection. Noises that may be heard include:

- Wheezing heard on expiration and indicating lower airway obstruction;
- Stridor heard on inspiration and indicating upper airway obstruction;
- Coarse crackles, indicating secretions;
- Fine crackles, indicating pulmonary oedema;
- Grunting heard on expiration in infants.

Palpation

The chest should be palpated to feel for any deformity. The fingers should be placed around the chest to feel if air entry is symmetrical and if there are any extra movements.

Percussion

Percussion is used to assess the areas of the lungs for consolidation. The correct technique is to hyperextend the middle finger of one hand and place the distal interphalangeal joint firmly against the child's chest. With the end (not the pad) of the opposite middle finger, use a quick flick of the wrist to strike the first finger. The sound made should be categorized as normal, dull or resonant. The front and back of the child's chest should be percussed.

Signs of respiratory distress

Respiratory distress is frightening for both the child involved and the family. It is important that interventions are fully explained to ensure that both the child and family are compliant with the required treatment.

Signs of respiratory distress include:

- Increased respiratory rate and depth
- Recession – subcostal, supraclavicular, tracheal tug
- Nasal flaring
- Grunting in infants during expiration
- Head bobbing – in older children
- Stridor or wheeze.

The signs of respiratory distress are related to the increased effort the body makes to try and improve gaseous exchange. Recession is characterized by the indrawing of the intercostal muscles in the chest and is seen most commonly in infants but can be seen in older children. Nasal flaring can be seen in most age groups and is a physiological response to try and increase the airway diameter. Grunting is heard in infants and is caused by the premature closure of the larynx. This is an attempt by the body to increase the infant's functional residual capacity (FRC; the amount of air left in the lungs at the end of expiration). By increasing FRC it becomes easier to reinflate the lungs during the next breath. The grunting noise is generated as air being exhaled hits the larynx as it has closed more quickly than normal. Head bobbing which is seen in older children, mainly toddlers, is the result of sheer physical effort: as they take a breath in they pull down so hard that their head bobs down and then up again as they relax during exhalation.

Stridor is heard on inspiration and is caused by upper airway obstruction. Wheeze is heard on expiration and is caused by lower airway obstruction. Other signs to look out for are the child being unable to talk, a child who is very still and a child who was very distressed but becomes passive. These are all signs of worsening respiratory distress as the child tries to conserve energy for breathing.

Respiratory investigations

Peak flow

Peak flow is a measure of peak expiratory flow. It is commonly used in children with asthma. It is a measure of the fastest rate at which air can be exhaled from the lungs. To predict normal peak flow for a child their height must be measured and plotted along with the peak flow on a chart called a nomogram. If the child is very distressed them measuring peak flow can cause bronchospasm and should be avoided.

The procedure for measuring peak flow is as follows:

1. Move measurement bar on peak flow meter to zero.
2. Stand up if possible.
3. Hold meter horizontally.
4. Open mouth and slowly inhale as large a breath as possible.
5. Put mouthpiece on the tongue and seal with lips.
6. Blow out a short hard fast breath.
7. Relax and rest.
8. Repeat three times and record best reading.

Pulse oximetry

Pulse oximetry is widely used within healthcare settings, with the main aim being to detect hypoxaemia before it can be detected by sight or before obvious symptoms are displayed (Mathews 2005). The pulse oximeter provides continuous, non-invasive monitoring of the oxygen saturation in haemoglobin in arterial blood. Pulse oximetry only measures the extent to which haemoglobin is saturated with oxygen and does not provide information on oxygen delivery to the tissues or ventilatory function (Higgins 2005).

The pulse oximeter consists of two light-emitting diodes (one infrared and one red) on one side of the probe. These transmit red and infrared light across the tissue bed (usually finger or toe), to a photo detector on the other side of the probe (Welch 2005). The ratio of absorption is relative to the concentration of oxygenated haemoglobin to deoxygenated haemoglobin (Chandler 2000). The more oxygenated the blood, the more red light passes through. By calculating the ratios of red to infrared light over time, oxygen saturation is calculated (Giuliano 2006).

The normal range for children (other than those with a known cardiac aetiology or chronic lung disease) is >95% (Fox 2002; Booker 2004). There are many different probe types used in practice. Common sites in children include:

- Finger or toe (using self adhesive probe or finger probe)
- The ear lobe (using clip probe)
- Across the palm of the hand (in smaller children)
- Across the foot (in smaller children).

An important point is that the area utilized should be cleaned and nail varnish removed to ensure accuracy of readings (Whaley and Wong 1999). The infrared light should shine down through the skin and on the opposite side the photo detector should be able to pick up a reading. The pulse oximeter screen should display a wave with a numerical reading at the end. If there is no wave form, the reading will not be accurate (this may be seen with poor tissue perfusion at the site used for measurement).

Other causes of inaccuracies with readings include:

- carbon monoxide poisoning whereby falsely high readings may be obtained;
- venous pulsation if the probe is secured too tightly or a blood pressure cuff is inflated above the probe site leading to a falsely low reading;
- factors that affect light absorption such as skin pigmentation, dried blood and intravenous dyes;
- patient movement such as shivering can lead to a falsely low reading or a inaccurate reading due to a poor trace;
- oxygen saturations less than 70% are unable to be accurately measured through pulse oximetry (Schnapp and Cohen 1990).

Probe sites should be changed frequently in practice as it has been documented that children may experience pressure sores and even superficial burns when probes have been left in situ for long periods. Best practice is to change them 4–6 hourly. Always note the use of supplementary oxygen when recording pulse oximetry and ensure an accurate trace is obtained when taking readings. Be aware of the effect that movement can have, particularly when dealing with children, and ensure that you observe skin colour and pallor alongside pulse oximeter readings. Observational assessment provides information on the accuracy of the pulse oximetry reading and must be considered when interpreting oxygen saturation levels.

Other investigations

Chest x-ray is commonly used in children with respiratory disease to establish if there are any areas of abnormality on the lung.

Microbiology is used to establish whether any sputum samples contain bacteria and which antibiotics they are sensitive to.

Virology is used in the diagnosis of bronchiolitis to ascertain if the child is RSV positive.

Blood gases are often used to assess children with acute respiratory problems. These are covered in detail in Chapter 3.

Respiratory interventions

There are several respiratory interventions that are used for children with different types of respiratory disease.

Oxygen administration

Oxygen is commonly used for children with respiratory disease. It is important that the correct method of administration is chosen both for the age and condition of the child. The child will also need monitoring with pulse oximetry and regular respiratory assessment if they are receiving oxygen. You should also record the amount of oxygen being delivered to the child, either in litres per minute or as a concentration – FiO_2. Oxygen should be regarded as a drug and should therefore be prescribed on the drug prescription chart (BMJ Publications 2006).

Factors to take into consideration when choosing oxygen delivery method:

- age of child
- clinical condition of child
- percentage/flow rate of oxygen prescribed
- compliance of child.

There are some complications that can occur when administering oxygen to children and these need to be taken into consideration. They are usually related to suboptimal delivery and monitoring techniques (Pease 2006). It is important to ensure that monitoring is reliable and accurate as this is being used as a method to assess the effectiveness of the oxygen therapy. Prolonged use of dry oxygen at high flow rates can cause drying of the mucous membranes which can lead to discomfort for the child. Oxygen toxicity can also be a problem and is caused when high levels of oxygen are delivered unnecessarily. The oxygen flow or concentration should be titrated to achieve a normal oxygen saturation of 95%. Care must also be taken when administering oxygen to children who may normally have a lower oxygen saturation level such as children with chronic airway disease or cardiac disease. It is important to establish what a normal saturation level is for these children and titrate the oxygen to achieve this. Artificially increasing the oxygen saturation level can be very dangerous for such children.

Nasal cannulae

Nasal cannulae are useful for infants who are obligatory nose breathers or for older children when a high percentage or fast flow of oxygen is required. Cannulae can deliver up to 2 litres per minute. They allow the child to feed and still receive oxygen. Humidification is not necessary as the gas is entering via nasal passages where it is warmed and moistened Ill-fitting cannulae can obstruct the nostrils so care needs to be taken that the correct size is chosen. They should occupy less than half the space in the nasal passage. Care also needs to be taken to ensure that the nostrils and the face do not become sore from the cannula. There is limited oxygen delivery available with this method, with the child receiving about 28% FiO_2 (Field 2005) when 2 litres per minute is delivered through the device.

Head box

Head boxes are very useful for delivering high concentrations of oxygen to infants. They can reliably deliver oxygen concentrations of up to 90%. They also provide high humidity as the oxygen must be humidified and warmed prior to it entering the head box. This is important as the temperature of the infant can be compromised if the oxygen is not warmed. The oxygen concentration in the head box can be monitored so allowing accurate recording of how much oxygen the infant requires. An oxygen analyser should be placed inside the head box to provide accurate measurement of the concentration of oxygen delivered to the child. It is very important that the opening of the head box where the infant is positioned is not obstructed in any way. Obstruction can lead to a build-up of exhaled carbon dioxide in the box and thus a decrease in oxygen concentration. The disadvantages of a head box are that the infant can be difficult to observe and it can create a barrier between infant and parents. The infant also needs to lie relatively still within the box. The infant will need to be removed for oral feeding and care, so it can be difficult to maintain a consistent level of oxygenation.

Simple face mask

This device delivers approximately 35–60% FiO_2 with a flow rate between 6 and 12 litres per minute (a minimum flow of 6 litres per minute should be maintained to prevent rebreathing of exhaled carbon dioxide). By utilizing elephant tubing, water and a heater, humidification can be achieved via this device. The insertion of an oxygen flow meter can also control the percentage of oxygen delivered and assist the practitioner in assessing the amount of oxygen required for the child to maintain normal or improved oxygen saturations. The mask should be the correct size to ensure a good fit, enabling optimum oxygen delivery. The mask comes in two sizes, paediatric and adult, and is therefore not appropriate for infants and smaller children. Rebreathing of CO_2 does occur with this device and the amount of oxygen received by the child is dependent on their respiratory effort, particularly the rate and tidal volume. Indications for this device may be simple postoperative recovery and short-term use.

Non-rebreathe masks with reservoir bags

This is a facemask with a reservoir bag attached. There are either one or two valves over the exhalation ports on the mask, allowing approximately 95–100% FiO$_2$ to be delivered. To achieve this the reservoir bag is connected to an oxygen supply, usually delivered at 15 litres per minute, which causes it to inflate and fill. The reservoir has a valve preventing exhaled air from entering and blocking entrainment of gas from the atmosphere on inspiration, ensuring that only supplemental oxygen contained within the reservoir bag is inhaled by the patient. Exhaled gas is directed out from the side ports on the mask. Oxygen delivered cannot be humidified and therefore drying out of the oral/nasal pharynx will occur. However, this device should be used as a short-term adjunct to oxygen delivery and the child must have continuous respiratory assessment if requiring this level of supplemental oxygen. Medical staff must be alerted to the amount of FiO$_2$ delivered to maintain normal oxygen saturations. It may be necessary for further respiratory support to be instigated (such as non-invasive ventilation).

Humidification

Humidification is important in the delivery of oxygen, primarily because it prevents the mucous membranes from drying out. Any oxygen that is going to be delivered for longer than 6 hours should be humidified. There are various methods by which the oxygen can be humidified. Different connectors are available from manufacturers that enable the oxygen delivery system to be connected to a disposable water bottle. The nasal cannulae connection is a simple snap-off valve that enables the cannulae to be connected directly to the water bottle. There are also adaptors available that allow the delivery of oxygen as a percentage. These are usually used with elephant tubing. It is important to follow the manufacturer's instructions and change the water delivery bottles at regular intervals. This is to prevent infection. The normal period of use is 24 hours. Most humidification systems also allow the oxygen to be warmed. This is important if the child is going to receive the oxygen for a prolonged period of time.

Suctioning

Suctioning is often required for children with respiratory disease. The procedure needs to be carried out with as little distress to the child as possible. Suctioning can be traumatic for children but it can also cause clinical distress with decreased oxygen saturations and increased work of breathing. Tables 4.2 and 4.3 list the procedures for oral and nasal pharyngeal suctioning.

Indications for suctioning

- The child's breathing becomes difficult due to vomiting or excessive secretions in the oral or nasal pharynx.
- The secretions are seen, heard and felt. Frothing or bubbling may be seen from the nose or mouth. Wet crackles maybe felt by placing a hand on the child's chest.
- The child's skin may look pale, blue or grey, particularly around the mouth or nose.
- The child is coughing excessively and unable to clear their secretions.

Table 4.2 Procedure for oral pharyngeal suctioning.

Action	Rationale
Explain procedure to the child and family	To ensure you gain consent and the child and family are prepared
Ensure you use universal precautions	To prevent spread of infection
Select the correct sized Yankauer/suction catheter	To reduce the risk of mucosal trauma
Check the suction machine is set to the correct pressure, 60 to 120 mmHg	To reduce the risk of mucosal trauma
Insert the catheter into the mouth, apply suction and remove secretions, ensuring the catheter does not go right to the back of the throat	To reduce the risk of mucosal trauma and prevent gagging
Repeat until all the secretions are clear	
Monitor the child's respiratory status throughout the procedure	To observe and treat deterioration quickly
Clean the suction catheter and tubing with water	To dislodge any secretions caught in the tubing
Ensure the child is comfortable	

Table 4.3 Procedure for nasal pharyngeal suctioning.

Action	Rationale
Explain procedure to the child and family	To ensure you gain consent and the child and family are prepared
Ensure you use universal precautions	To prevent spread of infection
Select the correct sized Yankauer/suction catheter the catheter should be no greater than 2/3 the diameter of the child's nostril	To reduce the risk of mucosal trauma and to ensure the child still has space to breathe around the catheter
Check the suction machine is set to the correct pressure, 60 to 120 mmHg	To reduce the risk of mucosal trauma
Insert the catheter into the back of the nose until the child coughs, remove the catheter, applying suction. This should take no longer than 2 to 3 seconds	To reduce the risk of mucosal trauma and oxygen deprivation
Repeat until all the secretions are clear	To observe and treat deterioration quickly
Monitor the child's respiratory status throughout the procedure	
Clean the suction catheter and tubing with water	To dislodge any secretions caught in the tubing
Ensure the child is comfortable	

Non-invasive ventilation

Non-invasive ventilation is now used more frequently in high dependency units. It can be used in a number of ways: to prevent a child needing intubation, to help wean a child from full ventilation and to provide respiratory support to children who have certain clinical conditions such as neuromuscular disorders or cystic fibrosis.

Non-invasive ventilation has different modes of delivery. It can be delivered to infants and children using masks, a flow driver or a cuirass. Masks can be used to deliver two types of ventilation: continuous positive airway pressure (CPAP) and biphasic positive airway pressure (BIPAP). CPAP works by providing the child with a flow of gas at a set pressure. The child does the work of breathing, the in and out part, and the CPAP delivers some extra pressure (Killick 2001). CPAP has several benefits and is an effective way of delivering ventilatory support to both infants and older children.

The benefits of CPAP include the following:

- It increases functional residual capacity and alveolar recruitment.
- It promotes alveolar stability and reduces intrapulmonary shunting.
- It improves stability of large and small airways.

- It improves the rhythmicity of breathing, reducing apnoeic episodes.
- It decreases pulmonary vascular resistance.

For infants CPAP is delivered using a flow driver. The flow driver uses fluidic flip technology that deflects the flow of gas during exhalation, so that the infant does not have to exhale against an incoming flow of gas. CPAP is administered to the baby using short nasal prongs or a nose mask. In order to prevent excoriation of the nasal septum, nose care should be carried out at least 4-hourly, ensuring that there is no sign of skin breakdown. For infants who develop a sore nasal septum or for whom it is difficult to maintain an adequate seal with prongs, a nasal mask may provide relief. Prongs and masks are available in different sizes and it is important that the correct size is used. CPAP hats are also available in different sizes and these should be fitted carefully to ensure a good seal is achieved without causing too much pressure. As CPAP has a tendency to force gas into the oesophagus as well as the trachea, babies should always have an orogastric tube in situ to aid in decompression of the abdomen.

CPAP is delivered to older children using a specially designed face mask which is strapped onto the child's face to ensure a good seal.

BIPAP is delivered in the same way as CPAP via a face mask. The difference with BIPAP is that the pressure support provided can be timed to synchronize with the child's own breathing pattern (Preston 2001). This means that when the child starts to inhale to take a breath the machine will 'cut in' and provide some extra pressure support for that breath. The machine will then provide CPAP on expiration, so helping to stop premature airway closing and make the next breath easier for the child. Oxygen can also be delivered if the child requires it.

A cuirass is an externally fitted jacket that works by helping the chest wall to expand. It provides a negative pressure around the chest and this aids chest expansion. It leaves the mouth free so the child can feed normally when it is in situ (Klonin *et al.* 2000).

Non-invasive ventilation has some physiological benefits over intubation and invasive ventilation. It mimics normal breathing, it allows communication and feeding, and it requires minimal or no sedation for the child to co-operate with its use.

Nursing interventions for children receiving non-invasive ventilation

Children receiving non-invasive ventilation need to have close observation of their respiratory status. They will need to have pulse oximetry monitoring and regular observation of their respiratory rate and heart rate. Close observation of the work of breathing and their colour and general appearance is also important. Care must be taken to ensure that their skin is observed, particularly if they are using a face mask or nasal prongs or mask. The skin can become sore and excoriated around this area so careful observation and skin care interventions are required. Mouth care is essential and careful note of the child's fluid input and output is required.

Positioning

Optimal positioning of children and infants can improve oxygenation and decrease respiratory workload (Wells *et al.* 2005). Positions that can improve work of breathing include:

- prone positioning
- sitting upright
- lying over someone's shoulder.

When caring for a child with respiratory distress it is important to consider the optimal position for them. Older children may find it easier to be sitting upright or to lean forward over a table or pillow. It is important that you regularly change the position of the child and that the effect of the position on the clinical condition of the child is assessed. The position should be recorded and the length of time the child has spent in the position should also be recorded.

Infants have better oxygenation when placed in the prone position but the difference is small (Wells *et al.* 2005). It is very important to emphasize to parents that prone positioning for infants must only be used in the hospital setting and when the infant is receiving continuous cardiovascular monitoring. This is due to the increased risk of sudden infant death that is associated with prone positioning.

Tracheostomy care

A tracheostomy is the formation of an opening into the trachea, usually between the second and third rings of cartilage. It provides a channel for effective respiration and for the removal of tracheobronchial secretions (Wilson 2005).

Indications for tracheostomy formation include:

- Long-term weaning from mechanical ventilation following critical illness;
- Protection of the tracheobronchial tree in conditions which may lead to aspiration, e.g. an unconscious patient;
- Conditions leading to respiratory insufficiency, e.g. neuromuscular disorders;
- Relief of respiratory obstruction, e.g. congenital abnormality.

For the child with a tracheostomy, breathing is dependent on the maintenance of a patent tube. However, the stoma also comprises several functions of the upper respiratory tract, including:

- Humidification and warming of inspired air.
- Filtering and cleansing of inspired air.
- Protection of the airway by the cough mechanism.

The size and type of tracheostomy tube to be used is decided by the surgeon who will be fitting it. If the tracheostomy is undertaken in an emergency situation then a standard basic tube will be used and this can be changed later if the tracheostomy needs to be kept for longer. The choice of tube is dependent upon the child's upper airway anatomy, physiological requirements and body size (Abraham 2003). Different types of tracheostomy tube include plastic and metal, cuffed and uncuffed, and fenestrated. Fenestrated tubes have a hole in the cannula which facilitates speech. Cuffed tubes are not normally used in children as their cartilage, muscles and mucous membranes are softer than an adult's. The lumen of the trachea is narrow and cuffed tubes can cause long-term damage and stenosis. This is to be avoided (Wilson 2005).

The tracheostomy tubes used for children are usually plastic and for small children uncuffed. The tube has three different components: the cannula which is the curved part that fits into the tracheal stoma, the neck flange which is the part of the tube that rests upon the child's neck, and the hub which is a 15 mm connector that allows attachment to a ventilator or other respiratory equipment. The flange has two holes on either side that allow a holder to be threaded through. The holder goes around the child's neck and is usually secured with Velcro.

Plastic tracheostomy tubes are sterile and are designed for single use. The tube is supplied with a smooth introducer that fits inside it and allows easy insertion of the tube into the tracheal stoma. The introducer should always be kept by the child's bedside in case it is needed to replace the tube in an emergency.

Nursing interventions required for a child with a tracheostomy

The priority when caring for a child with a tracheostomy is the safety of the child. It is vital that the nursing staff caring for the child are confident in the care of the tracheostomy and versed in emergency procedures. Each child needs to have the following equipment readily available at their bedside. This is to ensure the tube can be replaced in an emergency and tracheal suctioning can be carried out swiftly if required:

- Operational oxygen with a tracheostomy mask
- Operational suction
- Correctly sized suction catheters
- Spare tracheostomy tube of the correct size and also a tube one size smaller
- Equipment for universal precautions
- Lubricant
- Tracheostomy holder.

Nursing care for a child with a tracheostomy has the following components:

- Suctioning
- Cleaning the stoma
- Changing the holder
- Changing the tube (Wilson 2005).

Suctioning

Suctioning the tracheostomy is an intervention that is used frequently. It is similar to other suctioning techniques. It is required as having the tracheostomy prevents the patient from using their abdominal pressure to cough effectively and clear their secretions, and the tube itself causes irritation, so increasing the amount of secretions present (Hooper 1996). Multiple eye catheters have been shown to be more effective for suctioning (Day 2000) and research also shows that rotation of the catheter is not necessary (Day 2000). Humidification is important for a child who has a tracheostomy as the normal processes for warming and humidifying air are bypassed. Humidification can be provided y a Swedish nose (dry) or by oxygen if it is being administered (wet). Procedures for tracheotomy suctioning are given in Table 4.4.

Cleaning the stoma

The tracheal stoma site will need to be cleaned at least daily. The site initially is a surgical incision and is therefore at risk of infection. Once the site has healed then secretions can collect around the tube as it enters the stoma and on the skin surrounding it. The aim of cleaning is to keep the site clean and dry, therefore reducing the risk of infection and skin irritation. The site should be cleaned with 0.9% saline and a cotton wool applicator. Some centres use dressings around the stoma site, others do not. This is often down to the individual preference of the surgeon. Local Trust policies about the use and type of dressing should be followed.

Changing the tracheostomy holder

The holder or tapes securing the tube should be changed daily. Again the choice of securing device is variable by Trust. Some centres use

Table 4.4 Procedure for tracheostomy suctioning.

Action	Rationale
Explain procedure to the child and family	To ensure you gain consent and the child and family are prepared
Ensure you use universal precautions	To prevent spread of infection
Select the correct sized suction catheter	To reduce the risk of mucosal trauma
Check the suction machine is set to the correct pressure 60 to 120 mmHg	To reduce the risk of mucosal trauma
Insert the catheter into the tracheostomy 0.5 cm below the length of the tube, apply suction and remove secretions	To reduce the risk of trauma
Repeat until all the secretions are clear	
Monitor the child's respiratory status throughout the procedure	To observe and treat deterioration quickly
Clean the suction catheter and tubing with water	To dislodge any secretions caught in the tubing
Ensure the child is comfortable	

linen tapes and some use Velcro holders. If linen tapes are used they must be tied using a reef knot so that they can be undone quickly in an emergency. Whatever securing system is used, one finger should be able to be placed under the device to ensure that it is not too tight. The child's skin should be checked for redness and soreness and care should be taken to ensure that no pressure ulcers are developing.

Changing the tracheostomy tube

Tracheostomy tubes should be changed regularly to ensure that a build-up of mucus is not developing which could lead to respiratory distress and possible tube occlusion (Wilson 2005). Standard practice in many centres is to change the tube on a weekly basis (Wilson 2005) but care must be taken to ensure that the procedure is not carried out unnecessarily.

Factors that need to be taken into consideration when changing the tube include:

- Ensure the child has not just eaten, to prevent vomiting;
- Ensure the child is relaxed and, if likely to struggle, is held appropriately;
- Ensure all equipment required is to hand;

- Place a neck roll under the shoulders to allow the head to extend back providing a clear view of the stoma;
- Attach the holding device to the tube prior to insertion;
- Remove the old tube and place the new tube in situ immediately. Remove the introducer as the child's airway will be blocked while this is in situ;
- Secure the tube and suction the child if required;
- Oxygen may need to be administered.

Family support

Many children will be discharged into the community with a tracheostomy so a comprehensive plan of family education and support will be required. Families will need to be taught all the aspects of tracheostomy care and basic life support. Close liaison will be required between the community services and the hospital. Children should not be discharged until all the equipment required is at the home setting and the parents feel confident in their ability to manage the tracheostomy.

Intubation

Intubation may need to be undertaken in the high dependency unit. Staff should familiarize themselves with the equipment as the procedure will almost always need to be undertaken as an emergency.

The equipment required for intubation is listed in Table 4.5.

The procedure for intubation is as follows:

1. Open airway using chin-lift head-tilt.
2. Pre-oxygenate child using a self-inflating bag and 100% oxygen. Ensure oxygen saturation is above 95% before starting procedure.
3. Position patient into sniffing position.
4. Insert laryngoscope into mouth using left hand. Use suction if necessary.
5. Advance endotracheal tube through the cords.
6. Remove introducer.
7. Attach self-inflating bag, administer oxygen and check tube position by giving breaths and watching for chest movement and listening for air entry.
8. Secure endotracheal tube.

In emergency situations oral intubation is usually performed unless the medical personnel involved are very experienced. If this is the case then nasal intubation will be chosen as this is the preferred method for children.

Table 4.5 Equipment required for intubation.

Equipment	Size (if applicable)
Laryngoscope, curved or straight bladed	0–1 : neonate 1 : 6 months 1–2 : 1 to 2 years 2 : 4 to 6 years 2–3 : 6 to 12 years (4–5 : adult)
Endotracheal tube	Internal diameter (mm) = (Age/4) + 4 Length (cm) = (Age/2) + 12 for oral tube Length (cm) = (Age/2) + 15 for nasal tube
Magill forceps Suction source and catheters Self-inflating bag and mask Endotracheal tube introducer Tape to secure tube	 250, 500 and 1500 ml

Respiratory diseases

Asthma

Acute exacerbation of asthma is a major cause of admission of children to hospital. Asthma is characterized by reversible obstruction of both the large and small airways. Muscles of the bronchial tree become tight and the lining of the air passages swells, producing wheeze. Asthma is the most common chronic disease of childhood with approximately 1 million children suffering from asthma in the United Kingdom (Kissoon 2002). The airway obstruction is caused by an inflammatory reaction that may have an 'allergic' basis. Asthma is caused by a genetic predisposition combined with a viral infection and/or exposure to allergens such as house dust mite dander, tobacco smoke or environmental pollutants. The wheeze is heard on expiration as the trapped air is unable to leave the lungs. This results in the retention of carbon dioxide. In infants most wheezy episodes are caused by viral illnesses so it can be difficult to ascertain a diagnosis in the under-2 age group (Gallagher 2002). When making a diagnosis of asthma in children, the following clinical features are normally present:

- Personal history of atopic disease;
- Family history of atopic disease and/or asthma;
- A widespread wheeze is heard on auscultation;

- A history of previous episodes which improved with treatment;
- More than one of the following symptoms is present:
  - wheeze
  - cough
  - dyspnoea
  - chest tightness;
- These symptoms are frequent, recurrent, worse at night and in the early morning, occur in response to or are worse after exposure to exercise, cold air, pets or emotions.

Symptoms of an acute episode of asthma include: wheezing, cough, shortness of breath, increased work of breathing, cyanosis, anxiety and chest pain. Acute exacerbation of asthma can be categorized into different degrees of severity (Table 4.6). The treatment of asthma is related to the severity of the exacerbation (Table 4.7).

For children with life-threatening asthma, if there is no improvement then intravenous salbutamol should be considered. This requires a loading dose of 15 µg/kg over 10 minutes followed by an infusion of 1–5 µg/kg/min. ECG monitoring must be used for children receiving IV salbutamol as it can cause cardiac arrhythmias.

Nebulizers are only required for children with severe/life threatening asthma. The nebulizer converts the liquid medication into a fine mist and distributes it along the tracheobronchial tree. A mouthpiece or facemask can be used and the oxygen flow rate needs to be 6 to 8 litres per minute. The drug is usually delivered if the child is breathing normally within 10 minutes.

Table 4.6 Asthma: levels of severity. Adapted from British Thoracic Society (2008).

Moderate	Severe	Life threatening
$SpO_2 \geq 92\%$	$SpO_2 \leq 92\%$	$SpO_2 < 92\%$
Peak flow ≥50% best/ predicted (>5 years)	Peak flow <50% best/ predicted (>5 years)	Peak flow <33% best/ predicted (>5 years)
Able to talk	Too breathless to talk	Silent chest
Heart rate:	Heart rate:	Poor respiratory effort
≤130/min (2–5 years)	>130/min (2–5 years)	Agitation
≤120/min (>5 years)	>120/min (>5 years)	
Respiratory rate	Respiratory rate	Altered consciousness
≤50/min (2–5 years)	>50/min (2–5 years)	Cyanosis
≤30/min (>5 years)	>30/min (>5 years)	
	Use of accessory neck muscles	

Table 4.7 Treatment of asthma related to severity of exacerbation. Adapted from British Thoracic Society (2008).

Moderate	Severe	Life threatening
β2 agonist 2–4 puffs via spacer/ facemask	Oxygen via facemask	Oxygen via facemask Nebulized salbutamol 2.5 mg (2–5 years) 5 mg (>5 years) or terbutaline 5 mg (2–5 years) 10 mg (>5 years)
Consider soluble prednisolone 20 mg (2–5 years) 30–40 mg (>5 years)	β2 agonist 2–4 puffs via spacer/facemask or nebulized salbutamol 2.5 mg (2–5 years) 5 mg (>5 years) or terbutaline 5 mg (2–5 years) 10 mg (>5 years)	Ipratropium 0.25 mg
Increase β2 by 2 puffs every 2 mins up to 10 puffs according to response	Soluble prednisolone 20 mg (2–5 years) 30–40 mg (>5 years)	Soluble prednisolone 20 mg (2–5 years) 30–40 mg (>5 years) or IV hydrocortisone 50 mg (2–5 years) 100 mg (>5 years)
	Assess response to treatment 15 mins after β2	

Ongoing management of asthma

Ongoing management of asthma is very important to prevent life-threatening exacerbation and improve quality of life. The aims of ongoing management are to ensure that the child:

- Has no symptoms day or night
- Can play all sports and exercise
- Has minimal absences from school
- Has normal growth and development
- Requires a bronchodilator less than 3 times a week
- Has normal lung function (British Thoracic Society 2008).

Preventive measures that have been shown to be helpful in the control of asthma include:

- Breast feed for at least 4 months
- Don't keep furry or feathered pets
- Reduce exposure to house dust mite dander
- No smoking
- Reduce exposure to pollen (over 5s)
- Try to keep environment mould and damp free (British Thoracic Society 2008).

Prior to discharge home it is important that families and children understand the importance of preventive measures and also of taking their medication correctly Current guidance suggests that regular use of a steroid inhaler with intermittent use of a reliever is the preferred treatment regime for the majority of children. Inhaler technique should also be checked prior to discharge.

Bronchiolitis

Bronchiolitis presents with breathing difficulties, poor feeding, irritability, wheeze and, in the very young, apnoea. It is most common in infants aged 3 to 6 months (Scottish Intercollegiate Guidelines Network 2006). It is a seasonal disease which is more common in the winter months and it occurs in association with viral infections. The most common virus it is associated with is respiratory syncytial virus (RSV) which accounts for approximately 75% of cases (Greenhough 2002). RSV infection is very common with 70% of all infants being infected with it in the first year of life with 22% of these going on to develop bronchiolitis (Panitch 2001). Preterm infants are particularly vulnerable to the infection and often require hospital admission. Other vulnerable groups include infants with congenital heart disease and infants with chronic lung disease of prematurity. A diagnosis of bronchiolitis is made by using clinical symptoms. The first symptoms that appear are nasal discharge and a dry, wheezy cough.

Symptoms of bronchiolitis are:

- cough
- wheezing
- tachypnoea
- tachycardia
- recession
- nasal flaring
- poor feeding
- irritability
- apnoea
- crackles/crepitations.

Hospital admission is advised if the infant has the following symptoms and clinical signs:

- poor feeding (less than 50% of normal intake in the preceding 24 hours)
- history of apnoea
- lethargy
- grunting/nasal flaring
- respiratory rate of ≥ 70 rpm

- severe chest wall recession
- cyanosis (SIGN 2006).

Signs of a worsening clinical picture are failure to maintain oxygen saturations above 92% with an increasing oxygen requirement, deteriorating respiratory status and increasing respiratory distress and recurrent apnoea. In these circumstances then admission to HDU or PICU is recommended (SIGN 2006).

Fever is not always present. Investigations that should be undertaken include oxygen saturation monitoring and chest x-ray in severe cases. Rapid RSV testing is recommended so that isolation or cohort nursing can be instigated. No drug treatments have been found to be effective for bronchiolitis (SIGN 2006) so the management involves the use of supportive measures. These include oxygen therapy, suctioning, positioning and supplemental feeding. Nasogastric feeding or intravenous fluids are often required as the infant is particularly vulnerable to dehydration. Physiotherapy is not recommended. Saturation monitoring should always be used for these infants. RSV is very infectious so it is important to isolate the infant on admission once a diagnosis has been established so that infants who are RSV positive can be cohort nursed together.

There is an association between bronchiolitis and chronic respiratory symptoms. Infants are more likely to have recurrent wheeze and airway hyper-reactivity and to go onto develop asthma (Greenhough 2002).

Upper airway obstruction

Viral croup (laryngotracheobronchitis)
Viral croup is usually caused by parainfluenza. It is the most common cause of airway obstruction in young children. It occurs predominantly in infants (1–3 years) and is characterized by subglottic inflammation and narrowing (Bjornson and Johnson 2008). Oesophageal foreign body may present with similar symptoms, as can tonsillitis, so it is important that a history is taken to obtain the correct diagnosis. It is most common between October and March, but can occur at any time of the year and the symptoms are worse at night (Orlicek 1998).

Symptoms of viral croup include:

- barking cough
- coryzal symptoms
- stridor on inspiration
- signs of respiratory distress.

Management of croup involves keeping the child as calm as possible as anxiety can cause the symptoms to become worse. Steroids are usually used in a combination of nebulized and/or oral. Dexamethasone may be given orally at a dose of 0.6 mg/kg either as a one-off dose or for up to 3 days until symptoms have improved. Budesonide 2 mg is usually used, again as a one-off dose, but can be repeated after 30 to 60 minutes if clinically indicated.

Symptom progression is related to the level of stridor the child exhibits:

- Stridor on exertion > stridor at rest > recession on exertion > recession at rest > exhaustion, respiratory failure

In severe cases nebulized epinephrine can be used but ECG monitoring must be in place as this can cause severe tachycardia.

Epiglottitis

Epiglottitis is bacterial in origin, the causative agent usually being *Haemophilus influenzae*. It occurs in older children (3 to 6 years) and is relatively uncommon (Lerner and Perez Fontan 1998). It is however severe and life threatening. Placing the child in a supine position or extending the neck may precipitate acute obstruction and respiratory arrest.

Symptoms include:

- drooling
- sore throat
- difficulty in swallowing
- breathing difficulties
- stridor
- hoarseness
- fever and shivering
- cyanosis.

Extreme caution needs to be used when approaching the child and airway examination can cause complete obstruction. The airway needs to be secured, usually by intubation, and antibiotics are then used to treat the infection.

Foreign body inhalation

Foreign body inhalation can cause severe airway obstruction. The severity of the obstruction needs to be assessed and the appropriate action taken (see Figure 4.1).

Symptoms of foreign body inhalation:

- no history of preceding illness
- no fever
- sudden onset of stridor
- cough (bronchospasm as object reaches bronchial tree)

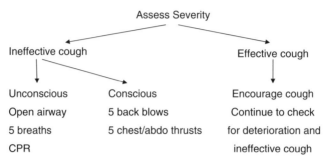

Figure 4.1 Management of child with inhaled foreign body.

- history of playing with small objects prior to onset of symptoms
- wheeze.

Management of foreign body inhalation involves removal of the object using a bronchoscope under general anaesthesia. Antibiotics may need to be given after the procedure.

Case study 1: 4-year-old with asthma

James is aged 4 and has suffered from asthma for two years. He has been admitted from A+E with an acute exacerbation of his asthma. On admission his observations are:

Respiratory rate 35 rpm, heart rate 100 bpm, temperature 37 °C, oxygen saturation 90% in 5 litres per minute of oxygen via a face mask.

Management

- What should your initial actions be?
    1. Complete ABC assessment.
    2. Check the time of last bronchodilator administration.
    3. Increase oxygen delivery and change to a rebreathe face mask.
- What monitoring does James require?
    1. James needs pulse oximetry and regular cardiovascular assessments to be undertaken.
    2. It would be inappropriate to undertake a peak flow at this time as it may worsen James' bronchospasm.

- What medication should be administered?
  1. β2 agonist 2–4 puffs via spacer/facemask or nebulized salbutamol 2.5 mg (2–5 years).
  2. Soluble prednisolone 20 mg (2–5 years).
- What would you do if the wheezing and respiratory distress do not improve?
  1. Repeat bronchodilator.
  2. Start cardiac monitoring.
  3. Consider ipratropium 0.25 mg.
  4. If no improvement then consider intravenous salbutamol.
  5. Blood gas measurements should be obtained.
  6. Close respiratory monitoring is essential.

Case study 2: 6-month-old with bronchiolitis

Ahmed is 6 months old. He is admitted to the high dependency unit with a suspected diagnosis of RSV bronchiolitis. On admission he has intercostal recession, nasal flaring and is grunting. His observations are:

Respiratory rate 80 rpm, heart rate 120 bpm, temperature 37.5 °C, oxygen saturation 89% in 2 litres per minute nasal cannula oxygen.

Management

- What should your initial actions be?
  1. Complete ABC assessment.
  2. Change oxygen delivery method to head box so that the concentration of FiO_2 can be increased and monitored until Ahmed's saturations reach a satisfactory level.
  3. Commence saturation monitoring.
- What monitoring does Ahmed require?
  1. Respiratory assessment.
  2. Cardiovascular assessment.
  3. Saturation monitoring.
  4. Blood gas analysis if his condition deteriorates.
- What would you do to meet Ahmed's nutritional needs?
  1. Establish normal feeding pattern. Is he breast or formula fed?
  2. Nasogastric tube should be passed if he is unable to feed normally.

3. Breast feeding should be maintained as it causes a lower drop in saturations than bottle feeding.
4. If Ahmed is unable to feed orally then either expressed breast milk or formula milk should be given via nasogastric tube.
5. Urine output needs to be monitored to ensure Ahmed is not dehydrated.
- What medication should be administered?
  1. No medication has been found to be effective in the treatment of bronchiolitis.
- What infection control procedures need to be implemented?
  1. Ahmed should be isolated or cohort nursed with other infants who are RSV positive.
  2. Universal precautions should be adhered to.

Conclusion

This chapter has examined common respiratory illnesses and the interventions and management required for them. Respiratory assessment and the identification of respiratory distress have also been discussed.

Learning activities

- Reflect upon the care you have provided for a child with asthma. How were their symptoms managed? What health promotion did you provide for them and their family?
- Reflect upon the care of an infant with bronchiolitis. How was feeding managed effectively for them?
- Think about caring for a child who has inhaled a foreign body. What health promotion discussions do you think would be suitable for the family?

References and further reading

Abraham S (2003) Babies with tracheostomies: the challenge of providing specialized clinical care. The ASHA Leader-online. www.asha.org/about/publications/leader-online/archives/2003/q1/030318

BMJ Publishing Group (2006) *British National Formulary for Children*. www.bnfc.org. BMJ Publishing Group/RPS Publishing/RCPCH Publications, London.

Bjornson C, Johnson W (2008) Croup. *Lancet* **371**: 329–339.
Booker R (2004) The effective assessment of acute breathlessness in a patient. *Nursing Times* **100**(24): 61.
British Thoracic Society Scottish Intercollegiate Guidelines Network (2008) *British Guideline on the Management of Asthma*. London.
Chandler T (2000) Oxygen saturation monitoring. *Paediatric Nursing* **12**(8): 37–42.
Day T (2000) Tracheal suctioning when why and how. *Nursing Times* **96**(20): 13–15.
Docherty B, Bench S (2002) Tracheostomy management for patients in general ward settings. *Professional Nurse* **18**(2): 100–104.
Field D (2005) Respiratory care. In Sheppard M, Wright M (eds) *Principles and Practice of High Dependency Nursing*, 2nd Edition. Elsevier, Edinburgh: 75–122.
Fox N (2002) Pulse oximetry. *Nursing Times* **98**(40): 65–67.
Gallagher C (2002) Childhood asthma: tools that help parents manage it. *American Journal of Nursing* **102**(8): 71–83.
Greenhough A (2002) Respiratory syncytial virus infection: clinical features, management and prophylaxis *Current Opinion in Pulmonary Medicine* **8**: 214–217.
Giuliano KK (2006) Knowledge of pulse oximetry amongst critical care nurses. *Dimensions of Critical Care Nursing* **25**(1): 44–49.
Higgins D (2005) Pulse oximetry. *Nursing Times* **101**(6): 34.
Hooper M (1996) Nursing care of the patient with a tracheostomy. *Nursing Standard* **10**(34): 40–43.
Killick L (2001) How To guides: Noninvasive ventilation in infants during interhospital transfer. *Care of the Critically Ill* **17**(5).
Kissoon N (2002) Acute asthma: under attack. *Current Opinion in Pediatrics* **14**: 298–302.
Klonin H, Bowman B, Peters M *et al.* (2000) Negative pressure ventilation via chest cuirass to decrease ventilator-associated complications in infants with acute respiratory failure: a case series. *Respiratory Care* **45**(5): 486–490.
Lerner D, Perez Fontan J (1998) Prevention and treatment of upper airway obstruction in infants and children. *Current Opinion in Pediatrics* **10**: 265–270.
Mathews PJ (2005) The latest in respiratory care. *Nursing Management Supplement: Critical Care Choices* **18**: 20–21.
Orlicek S (1998) Management of acute laryngotracheobronchitis. *Pediatric Infectious Disease Journal* **17**(12): 1164–1165.
Panitch H (2001) Bronchiolitis in infants. *Current Opinion in Pediatrics* **13**: 256–260.
Pease P (2006) Oxygen administration: is practice based on evidence? *Paediatric Nursing* **18**(8): 14–18.

Preston R (2001) Introducing non invasive positive pressure ventilation. *Nursing Standard* **15**(26): 42–45.

Schnapp LM, Cohen NH (1990) Pulse oximetry: uses and abuses. *Chest* **98**: 1244–1250.

Scottish Intercollegiate Guidelines Network (2006) *Bronchiolitis in Children: a national clinical guideline.* SIGN, Edinburgh.

Welch J (2005) Pulse oximeters. *Biomedical Instrumentation and Technology* March/April: 125–130.

Wells D, Gillies D, Fitzgerald D (2005) Positioning for acute respiratory distress in hospitalised infants and children. *Cochrane Database of Systematic Reviews* Issue 2. Art. No.: CD003645. DOI: 10.1002/14651858.CD003645.pub2.

Whaley L, Wong D (1999) *Nursing Care of Infants and Children,* 6th Edition. Mosby, Missouri, MO.

Wilson M (2005) Tracheostomy management. *Paediatric Nursing* **17**(3): 38–43.

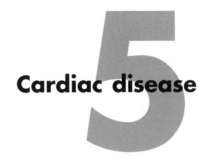

Cardiac disease

Andrea Cockett

Learning outcomes

- To develop an understanding of the two main types of cardiac disease that occur in childhood
- To develop an understanding of the assessment of children with cardiac disease
- To develop an understanding of the pathophysiology and management of cardiac failure
- To develop an understanding of nursing interventions for children with cardiac disease
- To develop an understanding of common arrhythmias and their management

Introduction

The aim of this chapter is to give an overview of cardiac disease in children. The anatomy and physiology of the cardiovascular system will be briefly described and assessment of children with cardiac disease will be covered. Cardiac disease will be discussed, as will cardiac failure which is the main presenting problem of cardiac disease. Finally, the most common arrhythmias and their management will be discussed.

Cardiac disease is relatively rare in general paediatric settings but it is important to have an understanding of it as children will often present at local centres prior to being transferred to a regional cardiac centre. There are two types of cardiac disease that present in childhood: acquired and congenital. Congenital is by far the most common. Both types of cardiac disease can present children with the same problem which is cardiac failure.

Cardiac anatomy and physiology

The heart is essentially a muscular bag. There are two chambers at the top of the heart, the atria, and two at the bottom, the ventricles. These chambers are connected by valves. The right atrium and ventricle are connected by the tricuspid valve and the left atrium and ventricle by the mitral valve. The blood flows into the heart via the superior and inferior vena cava and then travels through the right side of the heart via the pulmonary artery into the lungs to be oxygenated. The right ventricle is connected to the pulmonary artery by the pulmonary valve. Oxygenated blood leaves the lungs by the pulmonary veins and enters the left side of the heart, this then pumps blood around the body via the aorta. The left ventricle and aorta are connected by the aortic valve. The left and right atria are divided by the atrial septum and the left and right ventricles by the ventricular septum.

The heart has three layers of tissue. The innermost layer is the endocardium, which has a smooth surface to allow for the smooth flow of blood through the chambers of the heart. The middle layer is the myocardium. This is the muscular layer of the heart and makes up the bulk of the cardiac tissue. The outer layer is the epicardium. This consists of connective tissue and contains the blood vessels and nerves which supply the heart.

The heart itself is supplied by blood via the coronary arteries which branch off from the aorta just as it leaves the heart. Cardiac muscle combines the properties of the smooth muscle found in the lining of the gut, airways and blood vessels and the striated muscle of the muscoskeletal system. There are different types of cell found in the heart:

- myocytes or myocardial cells
- fibrous cells
- conducting cells.

Myocytes are specialized cardiac cells which provide the force needed to eject blood from the heart. The fibrous cells provide the connecting tissue of the heart and the conducting cells are responsible for the generation and conduction of the electrical signal required for contraction. Each of the cardiac cells is joined to the next by a specialized membrane called the intercalated disc. This is able to transmit both the force of the contraction and the electrical signals needed for conduction.

The heart is able to generate electrical activity of its own without any external stimulation, which allows contraction to take place. This is in the form of action potentials. However, the autonomic nervous system influences the rate of impulse generation, the depolarization and repolarization of the myocardium, and the strength of contractions. The impulse to beat is driven from the sinoatrial (SA) node which is located in the right atrium. Other cells have the potential to beat but the faster rhythm of the SA node is dominant. The SA node is the pacemaker of the heart. For a coordinated beat there has to be rapid impulse conduction and this is provided by the atrioventricular (AV) node and the Purkinje system.

The electrical conduction of the heart happens in four stages:

1. The sinus node fires and the electrical impulse spread across the atria. This results in atrial contraction (P wave).
2. On arriving at the AV junction the impulse is delayed, allowing the atria time to contract and eject blood into the ventricles.
3. The impulse is then conducted down to the ventricles through the bundle of His, right and left bundle branches and Purkinje fibres, causing ventricular depolarization and contraction (QRS complex).
4. The ventricles then repolarize (T wave) (Jevon and Ewens 2007).

The cardiac cycle has two components:

1. ventricular contraction systole
2. atrial contraction diastole.

These components are controlled by the conduction system. The cardiac cycle starts with ventricular systole. Pressure in the ventricles rises above atrial pressure and this causes the closure of the valves connecting the two chambers. Once pressure in the ventricles rises above arterial pressure the valves connecting the ventricles to the great vessels (aorta and pulmonary arteries) open. Blood is then ejected from the heart. As the aortic and pulmonary artery pressure rises the ejection of the blood then slows and stops. This ejection of blood causes the pressure in the ventricles to fall and the aortic and pulmonary valves then close. As this is happening the atria have filled and the valves between the atria and ventricles open again and the ventricle fills with blood ready to eject it and begin the cycle again.

Cardiovascular assessment

Presentation of cardiac disease

Neonates and infants present differently to older children. They may present with cardiac failure, cyanosis, collapse, weak femoral pulses and a heart murmur. They may also have other features not related to the cardiac problem, such as dysmorphic features and other congenital abnormalities. Neonates may present with abnormal weight gain in the first two weeks of life. It is physiologically normal for infants to lose and regain their birth weight in this period. If this does not happen, and weight gain is seen with other symptoms, this may indicate retention of fluid and a cardiac problem.

Older children may present with a murmur, heart failure, chest pain or palpitations. They can also present with unusual episodes in the case of arrhythmias and it can sometimes be difficult to differentiate between seizures and cardiac problems.

History

History taking is particularly important in cardiac disease to enable us to differentiate it from respiratory disease. Cardiac and respiratory disease can often present with similar symptoms, particularly in infants. History taking for cardiac disease has two components: the presenting complaint and the past history.

Presenting complaint:

- Is the onset sudden or has the child been unwell for some days?
- What symptoms is the child showing?
- Is there any chest pain?
- Has the child been feeding normally?
- Has there been any vomiting or loss of appetite?
- Has there been a fever?
- Has the child been able to exercise normally?

Unusual episodes can also be indicative of cardiac disease in infants and children, and these need to be assessed with a detailed history. Assessment of unusual episodes should include:

- Are the episodes precipitant, warned?
- What is the relationship to exercise, feeding and posture?
- Details of the attack such as onset, pain, palpitations, breathing, headache, giddiness or nausea?
- Cessation, if it is sudden or gradual, if there is a trigger, inducible?
- Is there a family history of episodes?

Once the history has been taken then the assessment of the cardio-vascular system can be undertaken.

Inspection

Inspection of a child with suspected cardiac disease should first involve looking for signs of cyanosis. Central cyanosis is a key feature of cardiac disease particularly some congenital defects. The altered blood flow patterns that exist in some congenital cardiac anomalies result in hypoxaemia that is visible as cyanosis. Cyanosis comes from the Greek *kuaneos* meaning blue. Cyanosis is a bluish colour of the nail beds, skin and mucous membranes and is produced by deoxygenated haemoglobin. The presence of cyanosis reflects hypoxaemia, a reduced arterial saturation (Horrox 2002). It also reflects hypoxia, a decrease in tissue oxygenation and impaired cellular processes due to low arterial saturations. Central cyanosis results from arterial desaturation and usually indicates cardiac or pulmonary disease. Assessment of cyanosis can be difficult. Visual assessment may not always be accurate and can be affected by the child's skin pigment, the quality of the light, the child's clothing and the colour of the room (Horrox 2002). Pulse oximetry is useful in determining peripheral saturation but must be used with caution as it is inaccurate at lower levels. Arterial blood gas analysis can be used but is an invasive test.

The respiratory system and chest should also be inspected. Is the chest a normal shape? An abnormal chest anatomy could indicate cardiac disease. Breathlessness is the commonest respiratory complaint with cardiac disease. The manifestation varies with age: infants present as poor feeders, older children present with decreased exercise tolerance. Stridor and wheeze can also be present. Orthopnoea can be reported by older children.

Oedema should then be observed for as it is a key feature of cardiac disease. In infants and small children oedema can be found around the eyes (periorbital), at the back of the neck and around the genitalia. In older children oedema is found around the dependent limbs. Weight should always be measured as abnormal weight gain is a sign of cardiac failure due to oedema.

Finally the features of the infant or child should be inspected. Infants with cardiac disease often have associated syndromes or other congenital abnormalities. The features should be inspected for dysmorphia and any other congenital defects such as cleft lip and palate should be noted.

Auscultation

Auscultation first involves listening to the apex beat. The practitioner is listening for rate and rhythm. Any extra or abnormal sounds should be noted and specialist advice sought. Murmurs are difficult to diagnose if the practitioner is not a specialist in the field. Normal heart sounds consist of:

- S1 first sound: This represents the closure of the mitral and tricuspid valves. Normally the two components cannot be heard separately.
- S2 second sound: This is produced by the closure of the aortic and pulmonary valves.
- S3 third sound: This is produced by the rapid filling of the ventricles during diastole. A loud third sound is normal in children.
- S4 fourth sound: This is also caused by ventricular filling during atrial contraction.

The respiratory system should be listened to at the same time. Wheeze and tachypnoea are very common in children with cardiac disease.

Palpation

Palpation is very important in a cardiovascular assessment. A central and a peripheral pulse should be checked. The practitioner is assessing for:

- rate
- rhythm
- volume.

The peripheral limbs should also be felt for temperature: are they warm and well perfused or are they cool and mottled? Blood pressure should be assessed; if cardiac disease is suspected then this should be a four-limb blood pressure with any differences between the limbs noted. If these are normal then one-limb blood pressure can be utilized. The liver and spleen should be palpated to look for enlargement as this is a sign of cardiac failure.

Percussion

Percussion should be used to assess the chest in the same way as for a respiratory assessment. It should also be used to assess the liver size. An enlarged liver is a sign of cardiac failure (Table 5.1).

Other investigations

ECG can be used for assessing rhythm, conduction disturbances, chamber enlargement, hypertrophy and strain.

Chest X-ray can be used to assess heart position, shape and size.

Table 5.1 Normal values of vital signs.

Age (mmHg)	Heart rate (awake)	Systolic BP (mmHg)	Diastolic BP (mmHg)	Mean BP (mmHg)
Newborn (3 kg)	100–180	50–70	25–24	40–60
Infant	100–160	85–105	55–65	50–90
Toddler	80–110	95–105	55–65	50–100
Preschool	70–110	95–110	55–65	50–100
School age	65–110	95–110	55–70	60–90
Adolescent	60–90	110–130	65–80	65–95

Echo cardiography provides a complete structural picture of the heart and the ability to measure pressure and blood flow within the heart.

Magnetic resonance imaging (MRI) provides a three-dimensional image of the heart.

Assessment of cardiac output

Assessing cardiac output is a key component of a cardiac assessment. Cardiac output is the amount of blood ejected from a ventricle per minute.

This is defined by two factors: the quantity of blood pumped by either ventricle during each beat (stroke volume) and the heart rate. Therefore:

cardiac output = stroke volume × heart rate

Stroke volume is the difference between end diastolic volume and end systolic volume:

stroke volume = EDV − ESV

End diastolic volume is determined by the length of ventricular diastole and the venous pressure. End systolic volume is determined by the arterial pressure in the aorta and pulmonary arteries before ventricular systole and the force of the ventricular contraction.

Cardiac output is therefore dependent on the following factors:

- preload
- contractility
- afterload
- heart rate and rhythm.

Preload is the amount of stretching of myocardial muscle fibres in response to variation in EDV before a contraction. It can be increased by manipulating the fibre length by increasing stroke volume with colloid, i.e. increasing venous return. This increased volume causes the muscle fibres to lengthen at the start of each contraction. Neonates however have a limited ability to do this due to the immaturity of the ventricular muscle mass.

Contractility is a measure of how efficiently the myocardial muscle fibres shorten. The force of contraction is reliant upon the length of the muscle fibres. The longer the fibre the more forceful the contraction. This theory is known as Frank-Starling's law.

Afterload is the resistance to ventricular ejection. It has two components:

1. The systemic vascular resistance which the left ventricle must overcome.
2. The pulmonary vascular resistance which the right ventricle must overcome.

Heart rate and rhythm are important in maintaining cardiac output as arrhythmias obviously affect the heart rate and decrease cardiac output. Temperature can affect the heart rate and decrease cardiac output and drugs can also affect heart rate and rhythm.

Blood pressure is also important in the assessment of cardiac output.

blood pressure = cardiac output × afterload

There is a detailed discussion of blood pressure in Chapter 3.

Assessment of cardiac output (Table 5.2) takes into consideration the signs and symptoms of cardiac failure.

Table 5.2 Factors considered in assessment of cardiac output.

	Low cardiac output	Adequate cardiac output
Peripheral perfusion	Poor	Good
Core–toe gap	>2 °C	<2 °C
Pulses	Impalpable or weak	Full
Urine output	<1 ml/kg/hr	>1 ml/kg/hr
Mental status	Combative, disorientated	Co-operative
Arterial pressure waveform	Small area under curve, dicrotic notch soon after peak	Large area under curve, dicrotic notch appears later
Metabolic acidosis	Base excess ≥5 mmol/l	Base excess ≤5 mmol/l

Cardiac failure

Cardiac failure is the inability of the heart to supply the body and the heart muscle itself with adequate circulatory volume or pressure (Shaddy 2001). It is the inevitable consequence of all forms of cardiac disease in children. The causes usually involve alterations of:

- contractility, the ability of the muscle to contract
- preload, the amount of blood returning to the heart
- afterload, the resistance to the ejection of blood from the heart
- the ratio of oxygen supply to demand.

The body produces a systemic compensatory response which leads to the signs and symptoms of cardiac failure. The sympathetic nervous system is stimulated and this leads to: increased heart rate, increased dysrhythmias, peripheral vasoconstriction, and mottled and cool skin. The renin-angiotensin mechanism in the kidneys is stimulated and this leads to sodium and water retention, oliguria, peripheral oedema and weight gain (fluid only). Systemic venous engorgement occurs due to stasis of blood and this leads to: increased liver size, jugular venous distension, peripheral or periorbital oedema, ascites and pleural effusion. Pulmonary venous engorgement occurs and this leads to tachypnoea, wheezing, increased respiratory effort, pulmonary oedema and central cyanosis. Not all of these symptoms will be present initially but will develop as the cardiac failure progresses. Children who present with acute sudden cardiac failure will show the majority of these signs.

Low cardiac output will be present in cardiac failure and this leads to the following symptoms:

- irritability
- poor feeding
- lethargy
- prolonged feeding with a poor suck
- tachycardia/gallop rhythm
- oliguria
- pallor
- peripheral cyanosis
- decreased capillary refill
- pulsus paradoxus.

Treatment of cardiac failure involves the management of the underlying condition that is causing the failure (Shaddy 2001). This will involve surgery for some children, drug therapy for others and in extremely severe cases transplantation (Westaby et al. 1999). Other interventions that are often required are:

Oxygen therapy

This is useful for some children with cardiac failure but must be used with caution in children with congenital cardiac disease. If the child's condition does not improve with oxygen therapy and you have no firm diagnosis then oxygen is probably contraindicated.

Nutritional support

This is often required either in the short term as nasogastric feeding or in the longer term as gastrostomy feeding.

Ventilation

Ventilation is often needed for children with acute severe cardiac failure.

Pharmacological management

The aim of pharmacological management is to improve the cardiac function and alleviate the symptoms of cardiac failure. Drug therapy involves the use of diuretics to relieve oedema, both systemic and pulmonary. A combination of potassium sparing and loop diuretics is used. Angiotensin-converting enzyme inhibitors are the cornerstone of treatment for cardiac failure (Westaby *et al.* 1999) and are used for the majority of such children.

Nursing interventions

Nursing interventions for children with cardiac failure focus on their symptoms and the monitoring and relief of symptoms.

- Try to improve cardiac output:
  - Increase oxygen supply by providing supplemental oxygen if appropriate and positioning for optimum oxygenation;
  - Decrease oxygen demand by maintaining normothermia, reducing activity, increasing calorie intake, nasogastric feeding, ventilation and if necessary sedation;
  - Administer prescribed medication and monitor its effectiveness.
- Observation of cardiac status:
  - Heart rate, temperature, capillary refill, respiratory rate
  - Four-limb blood pressure
  - Daily weight.
- Control fluid status:
  - Recording of input and output
  - Daily weight
  - Maintaining fluid restriction

- Pharmacological interventions
- Assessment and recording of oedema.

Management of chest drains

Chest drainage may be needed for children suffering with cardiac disease. They are also used for children who have respiratory problems. A chest drain is a one-way drain allowing fluid or air to be drained from the pleural cavity (Sullivan 2008). A chest drain in used when the child is suffering from any of the following problems:

- pnuemothorax
- haemothorax
- pleural effusion
- empyema
- chylothorax
- after cardiac surgery.

The chest drain allows for the reinflation of the lung, so improving the child's respiratory status. The drain may also be responsible for the removal of fluids such as blood, chyle or pus. The drain is normally inserted into the pleural cavity and consists of the drainage portion which enters the child's chest and a sealed bottle which contains a one-way system. The most commonly used type of drain is an underwater sealed drain. This is a bottle that consists of two chambers. One chamber contains water and stops air being able to enter the lung via the chest drain tube. The second compartment is where fluid from the pleural cavity drains into. This compartment allows the drainage fluid to be measured so that the child's fluid losses can be recorded, and replaced if necessary. The drain needs to be sealed with a one-way system so that air cannot enter the lung via the chest drain tubing and cause the lung to deflate.

Insertion of a chest drain

Insertion of a chest drain is a painful procedure and therefore before the insertion thought will need to be given to the level of analgesia and sedation required by the child. This will be dependent upon the age and clinical condition of the child. In ideal circumstances the procedure would be carried out with the child well sedated but this may not be possible if the child has a severe respiratory compromise. Adequate analgesia, both systemic and local to the insertion site, must be provided. Distraction techniques should also be utilized during the procedure to aid the child's coping mechanisms. The position of the drain in the chest is decided by the reason for insertion. If the drain is there for air removal then it is usually inserted in the apical area of the lung. If however the drain is there to drain fluid and air then it will be inserted into the base of the lungs. The child will need to be placed in the correct position for the different insertion locations. Insertion of the drain is an aseptic technique and the role of the nurse during insertion is primarily to monitor the child's condition during the procedure and, second, to aid the medical staff. Close observation will need to be made to of the child's cardiovascular and respiratory status. The child will also need to be closely monitored for signs of pain or distress. Once the drain is inserted the child and parents need to be informed about the care of the drain whilst it is in situ. The nursing care of a child with a chest drain can be divided into three distinct areas:

- care of the drain itself
- care of the insertion site
- care of the child.

Care of the drain
When caring for a child with a chest drain there are several areas of care that need to be addressed in relation to the drain itself. Care must be taken prior to insertion of the drain to ensure it is set up correctly with the correct volume of water in the underwater seal component. The drain will then need to be observed for bubbling, swinging and the volume of drainage. These observations will all need to be recorded, normally one or two hourly. Bubbling and swinging indicate that air is being removed from the pleural space. When the bubbling stops it should mean that all the air has been removed (Sullivan 2008). The drain must be positioned correctly at the bedside with the level of the drain always kept lower than the child's chest. The drain must also be placed in a stand so that it cannot be accidentally knocked over, so breaking the underwater seal. If the child wishes to move around then the drain should be placed in a suitable vehicle so that it is kept safe and the correct level form the child's chest is maintained. Special drain trolleys can be used but a toy pram is also suitable. When the child is in bed the drain tubing will need to be supported so that it doesn't drag down. The tubing can be quite heavy in relation to the child and if it is left unsupported it can pull on the insertion site, causing redness and pain. The drain bottle itself should be changed if it becomes too full of fluid or once a week as per the Trust's policy. The bottle is changed by clamping the drain and then transferring the tubing to a new prepared bottle. There should be no other reason for clamping a chest drain. Clamping has been shown to have a detrimental effect on

intrathoracic pressure, causing it to rise and increasing the risk of a tension pneumothorax (Sheppard and Wright 2006). The drain may need to be attached to suction immediately after insertion. Using low pressure suction on the drain can improve the removal of air and fluid. The suction pressure is normally set at 5 kPa so a special low pressure suction unit is required. The level should be recorded on the observation chart along with the other drain observations.

Care of the insertion site

The drain insertion site will need to be observed to ensure that it remains infection free. The drain is secured by a suture so care must be taken to ensure that the drain is not pulled. Normally a keyhole dressing is placed around the insertion site and this will need to be observed once a day for exudate and adherence. It should only be changed when necessary; if intact and clean the dressing should be left in situ.

Care of the child

Having a chest drain in place can be distressing and painful. Children need to receive adequate analgesia so regular pain assessment and administration of appropriate analgesia is required. They should be encouraged to mobilize as moving around will encourage lung expansion.

Removal of the chest drain

Chest drains are removed once all air has been removed from the pleural space and any drainage of fluid has stopped. Removal of the chest drain, like insertion, can be distressing for a child. Adequate preparation is required for the procedure. Normally a combination of opioid analgesia such as oral morphine and a sedative agent such as midazolam are required. The child and family will need a comprehensive explanation, and distraction techniques should be practised prior to the procedure. Removal of the drain is a two-person job. The drain has a securing suture and also a purse-string suture around the insertion hole so that air can be prevented from entering the chest once the drain is removed. One nurse is responsible for cutting the securing suture and pulling the purse-string suture closed. The other is responsible for removing the actual drain. The procedure is described in Table 5.3.

Once the chest drain is removed then the child can mobilize freely. Normally the child will have an x-ray after drain removal to ensure that there is no residual pneumothorax.

Table 5.3 Procedure for removal of a chest drain.

Action	Rationale
Explain procedure to the child and family	To gain consent and co-operation
Teach appropriate distraction techniques to the child and family	To gain co-operation, ease drain removal and minimize distress
Administer prescribed analgesia 30 minutes prior to the procedure	To ensure the child is adequately analgised
Prepare all equipment	To ensure all necessary equipment is available for the procedure
Administer prescribed sedative to the child	To ensure the child's distress is minimized and the child is cooperative
Remove the drain from suction if this is on	To reduce the risk of lung trauma during removal
Remove dressing from the chest drain	To visualize the insertion site
Identify holding and purse-string sutures	To ensure the correct sutures are cut
Cut the purse-string suture to a length of 5 cm	To ensure there is enough purse string suture to tie
Cut and remove holding suture	
Ask child (if age appropriate) to take 2 deep breaths and then hold their breath, or observe child's breathing and remove drain during expiration	To minimize the risk of air entering the pleural space
Remove drain by pulling slowly and steadily	To minimize trauma
Tie purse-string suture	To stop air entering the pleural space
Check wound site and apply dressing if required	To ensure wound remains free from infection
Dispose of all equipment appropriately	To maintain safety
Observe child for signs of respiratory distress, cardiovascular instability and pain	To ensure child recovers from the procedure

Cardiac disease

Acquired cardiac disease

There are three main types of acquired cardiac disease: Kawasaki disease, cardiomyopathies and cardiac infections.

Kawasaki disease

Kawasaki disease is an acute febrile illness that occurs in young children, commonly preschoolers (Maconochie 2004). This disease is more common in boys, and boys are more likely to die if they present with the disease. It was first identified in Japan and remains more common there. There are specific diagnostic criteria for Kawasaki disease, namely:

- Fever of 5 days or more.
- Presence of four of the five conditions below:
  - bilateral conjunctival infection
  - changes in the mucosa of the oropharynx
  - changes in the extremities.(desquamation)
  - polymorphous rash
  - cervical lymphadenopathy.

The cardiac complication of the disease is the development of aneurysms on the coronary arteries. This is due to inflammation of the arteries (Maconochie 2004). Death is caused by myocardial infarction. Up to 20% of untreated children present with aneurysms so echo cardiography should be performed on all such children to rule out an aneurysm.

Treatment of Kawasaki disease involves the administration of high dose aspirin, administration of intravenous gammaglobulins and, in very severe cases, cardiac transplantation.

Cardiomyopathy

Cardiomyopathy is a disease of the myocardium. It is responsible for approximately 1% of paediatric heart disease (Davies 2000).

There are different types of cardiomyopathy which present with differing symptoms and pattern of damage to the myocardium.

Dilated cardiomyopathy

Dilated cardiomyopathy is the commonest childhood cardiomyopathy. It is the commonest reason for new presentation of heart failure in infancy. Survival is 60% at 5 years (Davies 2000); 50% of deaths occur in first 3 months after presentation. The following structural changes occur in dilated cardiomyopathy:

- Increased left ventricular mass
- Normal or reduced left ventricular wall thickness
- Increased left ventricular cavity size.

These structural changes lead to congestive cardiac failure due to the poor function of the left ventricle. No specific cause has been identified in the majority of cases but there is a familial element to the disease with over 30% of diagnosed cases having a family member with an enlarged left ventricle. The children often present with myocarditis as the first sign of the disease. Treatment needs to be tailored to individuals but in most cases this means cardiac transplantation.

Hypertrophic cardiomyopathy

Hypertrophic cardiomyopathy (HCM) is characterized by an asymmetric or symmetric increase in the left ventricular wall thickness (McKenna and Behr 2002). This leads to the left ventricular cavity being reduced in size. A high proportion of cases are known to be caused by mutations in genes. It is thought that up to 1 in 500 of the United Kingdom population may be affected. HCM patients can have normal life span but there is always the risk of sudden death (McKenna and Behr 2002) (see Figure 5.1).

Restrictive cardiomyopathy
Restrictive cardiomyopathy is characterized by an inability of the myocardium to relax in diastole. This is very rare in childhood. The only real treatment option is transplantation and the outcomes are often poor.

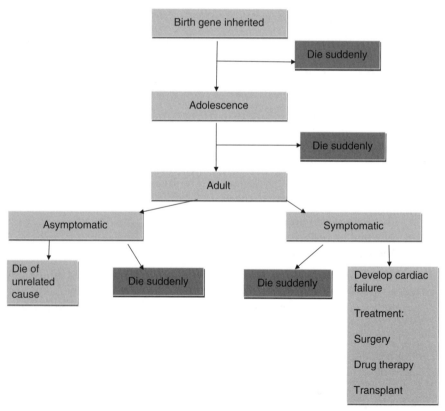

Figure 5.1 Natural histories of hypertrophic cardiomyopathy. Adapted from McKenna and Behr (2002).

Cardiac infections
Myocarditis
Myocarditis is inflammation of the myocyte (Hia *et al.* 2004). Viral myocarditis is the most common type but it can also be bacterial, fungal, parasitic or protozoal in origin. Myocarditis is the commonest cause of heart failure in previously healthy children.

Viral aetiologies:

* Enteroviruses (coxsackie virus) implicated in 25–40% of cases:
    * peaks in the spring and summer.
* Other viruses include:
    * cytomegalovirus
    * influenza
    * parainfluenza
    * mumps
    * measles
    * rubella
    * hepatitis C
    * HIV.

The virus enters the myocyte, replicates in the cytoplasm and leads to myonecrosis (Hia *et al.* 2004).

Chronic inflammation can occur due to the nature of the inflammatory response to the virus. Persistent viral infection is a predictor of poor outcome and progression to dilated cardiomyopathy. It is usually preceded by a respiratory infection (Leonard 2004).

Diagnosis – specific cardiac symptoms include:

* chest pain
* palpitations
* dyspneoa
* exercise intolerance
* hyperactive precordium
* quiet heart sounds
* tachycardia
* tachypnoea.

Treatment:

* Support cardiovascular function
* Intravenous immunoglobulin
* Steroids.

Survival:

* 86% at 1 month
* 79% at 2 years (Lee *et al.* 1999).

Endocarditis

Infective endocarditis is an infection of the lining of the heart, the endocardium and the heart valves (Prendergast 2004). Most cases of endocarditis in the developed world occur in children with congenital heart disease. It is most commonly caused by viridans streptococcus.

The onset is usually insidious, with general malaise, anorexia, arthralgia and fever. Mortality is high at around 20%. Treatment involves antibiotic therapy, usually of 4 to 6 weeks' duration (Prendergast 2004).

Congenital cardiac disease

Congenital cardiac disease (CCD) accounts for the majority of cardiac disease seen in children in the United Kingdom (Archer and Burch 1998). The incidence varies from 5/1000 to 8/1000 live births. Eighty percent of children present with the eight main defects but 32 different defects have been identified (Archer and Burch 1998). The cause of most congenital heart disease is unknown. There are some genetic causes that are known:

- Chromosomal, e.g. trisomy 21, Edwards syndrome, Turner syndrome;
- Single gene lesions, e.g. Noonan syndrome, Marfan syndrome;
- Contiguous gene lesions, e.g. Di George syndrome.

Some cases are linked to teratogens such as drugs and alcohol and some are linked to maternal diseases such as diabetes and lupus erythematosus.

Defects can be classified as:

- acyanotic defects
- cyanotic defects
- obstructive defects
- defects of mixed classification.

Neonatal presentation of congenital cardiac disease can be difficult to differentiate from other neonatal problems. Diagnosis can be difficult initially as the presentation can look like sepsis or respiratory distress. There are some diagnostic markers that differentiate CCD from the others:

- Central cyanosis if it is a cyanotic defect;
- The infant's condition is unresponsive to oxygen therapy;
- Cyanosis worsens with crying;
- Tachypnoea;
- The infant tires easily with feeding;
- Usually has a murmur;

- Usually has hepatomegaly
- Chest X-ray shows abnormally shaped or enlarged heart; there can also be a change in the pulmonary vascular markings.

Arterial blood gases are usually normal in acyanotic lesions while cyanotic patients have a decreased PaO$_2$. Blood chemistry is usually normal. Echo cardiography will obviously show the defect. To establish the presence of CCD, then 100% oxygen may be administered; if the PaO$_2$ remains below 20 kPa then the likely diagnosis is CCD. The management of the infant will depend on whether the defect is duct dependent or not and also on the condition of the child. If it is a duct-dependent defect then an infusion of prostaglandin E1 may need to be started to maintain duct patency. Intubation is not essential although it may be needed if the infant is acidotic prior to transfer to a children's cardiac centre. The most important management principle is to maintain a balance between pulmonary and systemic circulation. Oxygen is a pulmonary vasodilator and so causes a shift from systemic to pulmonary circulation.

This in turn will lead to systemic collapse if allowed to continue. Infants who show marked deterioration on oxygen, with a drop in cardiac output, should have the amount of oxygen being administered to them reduced to a maximum of 30%.

Nursing interventions for an infant with suspected congenital cardiac disease include:

- Maintenance of adequate tissue oxygenation by:
  - Observation of respiratory status;
  - Administration of a prostaglandin infusion E1 10 to 50 nanograms. Observation of side effects, apnoea, pyrexia, hypotension and seizures;
  - Administration of the minimum level of oxygen to maintain oxygenation.
- Potential for congestive cardiac failure:
  - Observe heart rate, blood pressure (in all four limbs);
  - Observe peripheral and core temperature;
  - Observe for oedema;
  - Observe peripheral perfusion.
- Potential inability to maintain normothermia:
  - Observe temperature, core and peripheral;
  - Nurse infant in a warming cot.
- Potential inability to maintain normal nutritional status:
  - Fluid is restricted to 50% of normal maintenance;
  - Until a firm diagnosis is made infants are normally kept nil by mouth;
  - Close observation of blood sugar needs to be made;

- Dextrose is usually used as maintenance to prevent electrolyte imbalances.
- Parental anxiety due to diagnosis.
  - Provide information;
  - Answer questions;
  - Inform parents of procedure for transfer to a regional referral centre.

The eight main cardiac defects will be discussed in this chapter.

Acyanotic defects
These are defects where the infant or child is not cyanotic. However, this does not mean the defect is not serious.

Atrial septal defect
Atrial septal defect is a hole in the septum, the muscular wall between the top two chambers of the heart, the right and left atria (see Figure 5.2). It occurs in 5 to 10% of children with a congenital lesion. It often happens in conjunction with other defects.
Presenting *symptoms*:

- This defect rarely presents with symptoms in infancy and is usually diagnosed antenatally or due to a murmur being detected during the infant's postnatal check.

Some ASDs close spontaneously without treatment (Horrox 2002). If the defect does not close spontaneously then it is usually closed by intervention. A small catheter is placed in the femoral vein and the catheter is passed up into the right atrium. A device is then released

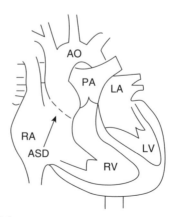

Figure 5.2 Atrial septal defect.

into the hole which blocks it off. The majority of defects are closed this way. Rarely, some children require cardiac surgery.

Patent ductus arteriosus

Patent ductus arteriosus (PDA) (Figure 5.3) occurs in 5 to 12% of children with congenital cardiac disease. It is more prevalent in preterm infants. The ductus arteriosus is a normal part of foetal circulation. It is a connection between the aorta and the pulmonary artery and it allows the shunting of blood away from the lungs of the foetus. In some infants the duct fails to close after birth. The closure of the duct is dependent upon the presence of specialized tissue which is present from 25 weeks' gestation and matures in the following 10 to 12 weeks of gestation. In term infants persistent patency is thought to relate to an anatomical defect in the specialized tissue.

PDA occurs in the following circumstances:

- As a single defect in preterm infants;
- As a single defect in term infants;
- In association with other cardiac defects;
- As a life-saving defect in some types of congenital cardiac defect where there is separation of the pulmonary and aortic blood flows and the patent duct provides the only flow of blood through the lungs (Horrox 2002).

Presenting symptoms (these are dependent on the size of the duct):

- Small duct:
  - murmur heard on examination.
- Medium duct:
  - cardiac failure
  - persistent respiratory infections

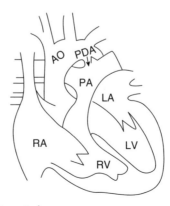

Figure 5.3 Patent ductus arteriosus.

- slow or below average weight gain
- increased respiratory rate
- large volume pulses.
- Large duct:
  - cardiac failure
  - breathlessness
  - poor feeding
  - poor weight gain
  - bounding pulses.

Treatment of a PDA depends upon the circumstances in which it occurs. Term infants are treated by device closure similar to that used for an ASD. Preterm infants are initially usually treated with drug therapy. Indomethacin is currently the drug of choice (Cooke *et al.* 2003). If this is not successful in closing the duct then surgery is used.

Ventricular septal defect
Ventricular septal defect (VSD) is a hole in the septum between the right and left ventricles (see Figure 5.4). It is the commonest cardiac lesion and accounts for approx 30% of all defects. It presents in infancy.

Presenting *symptoms* are again related to the size of the VSD.

- Small VSD:
  - murmur heard on examination.
- Medium VSD:
  - cardiac failure
  - persistent respiratory infections
  - breathlessness

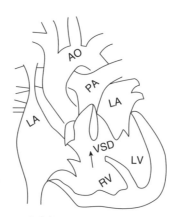

Figure 5.4 Ventricular septal defect.

- poor feeding
- poor weight gain.
- Large VSD:
  - cardiac failure
  - breathlessness
  - poor feeding
  - poor weight gain
  - grey colour
  - sweating
  - tachycardia
  - oedema.

Treatment can be interventional or surgical. Most commonly the hole is closed surgically but some cardiac centres are starting to close VSDs in the same way as ASDs.

Cyanotic defects
Tetralogy of Fallot
Tetralogy of Fallot (TOF) (Figure 5.5) is the most common cyanotic lesion and it accounts for 5 to 10% of all defects. It consists of:

- Ventricular septal defect;
- Pulmonary stenosis (narrowing of the pulmonary valve);
- Overriding aorta (where the aorta sits in between the right and left ventricles, taking blood from both. This means a mixture of oxygenated and deoxygenated blood enters the aorta);
- Right ventricular hypertrophy (thickening of the right ventricular wall).

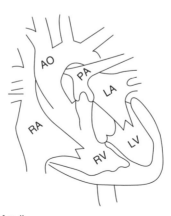

Figure 5.5 Tetralogy of Fallot.

The severity of the defect is based upon:

- The size and position of the VSD;
- The amount of obstruction of the pulmonary valve and artery.

Presenting *symptoms*:

- cyanosis shortly after birth when the ductus arteriosus closes
- cardiac failure
- breathlessness
- poor feeding.

One of the characteristic diagnostic features of TOF is 'spelling'. This is a sudden decrease in pulmonary blood flow. Spelling can be triggered by: crying, feeding and warm baths or beds which lead to vasodilation. The infant becomes hypercyanotic, pale, floppy and breathless. Spells are very dangerous so treatment must be instigated immediately. Treatment involves: putting the child in a knee to chest position, administering 100% oxygen, administering morphine and administering a beta blocker, usually propanolol.

Treatment of TOF involves surgical correction of the elements of the defect. This is usually carried out in the neonatal period. The VSD is closed and the pulmonary narrowing is corrected.

Transposition of the great arteries

Transposition of the great arteries (TGA) (Figure 5.6) is the second most common cyanotic defect. It is a duct-dependent defect which means the

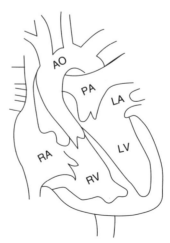

Figure 5.6 Transposition of the great arteries.

infant is entirely dependent on a patent ductus arteriosus for their systemic and pulmonary blood flow. The defect is characterized by the aorta and pulmonary arteries being in an incorrect anatomical position.

Presenting *symptoms*:

- Worsening cyanosis as the ductus arteriosus closes following birth
- Breathlessness
- Metabolic acidosis.

Initial *treatment* is focused around maintain the patency of the ductus arteriosus. This is achieved by the administration of a prostaglandin (prostin) infusion. The infusion is started immediately a diagnosis of TGA is made. The normal dose range is 0.05 to 0.1 microgram per kilogram per minute (Fleiner 2006). Side effects of prostin include apnoea, high temperature and arrhythmias so the infant needs careful monitoring (Hudspeth and O'Toole 2000). Surgical correction is usually carried out in the first week of life using a procedure known as a 'switch' operation (Hudspeth and O'Toole 2000). In this procedure the aorta and pulmonary artery are 'switched' back to their correct positions.

Obstructive defects

Coarctation of the aorta

Coarctation of the aorta (Figure 5.7) is a narrowing of the aorta. It is more common in boys, and infants can present in a state of collapse (Westmoreland 1999). The narrowing causes reduced blood flow to the lower half of the body.

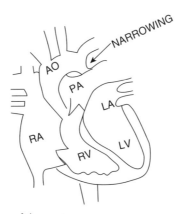

Figure 5.7 Coarctation of the aorta.

Presenting *symptoms*:

- Metabolic acidosis
- Absent femoral pulses
- Reduced blood pressure in lower limbs
- Collapse.

Treatment is by surgical correction. The most popular technique is known as end-to-end anastomosis where the narrowing is removed and the two ends are joined together.

Aortic stenosis
Aortic stenosis accounts for 5% of all defects. It is characterized by a narrowing of the aortic valve. It is more common in boys and can present in the neonatal period as critical aortic stenosis. It can be treated either surgically or interventionally (neonatal choice). The interventional approach involves inflating a balloon in the valve to stretch it open.

Pulmonary stenosis
Pulmonary stenosis accounts for 5 to 10% of all defects. It is characterized by a narrowing of the pulmonary valve. It can present in the neonate as critical and is usually treated interventionally in the neonate. Older children are treated surgically.

Arrhythmias
Arrhythmias can have many different causes. They are an abnormality in the rate, regularity or site of origin of the cardiac impulse. The most common causes include:

- hypoxia
- hypovolaemia
- low cardiac output
- hypothermia
- electrolyte imbalance
- acid–base abnormality
- cardiac abnormality
- infection
- hormonal disturbance
- neurological dysfunction
- drugs
- toxins.

When presented with a child having an arrhythmia it is important that a 12-lead ECG is recorded as this enables the correct diagnosis to be made. When interpreting an ECG the following factors need to be looked at: the rhythm, the rate, the QRS complex and the atrial activity.

The rhythm
When looking at the rhythm there are several elements of the ECG that need to be analysed to ensure the correct diagnosis is made. The R-R interval should normally be less than 0.12 seconds, the P-P interval should be regular, and any early or delayed beats should be noted. Any patterns of irregularity should be examined to see if they are repeated or chaotic.

The rate
The rate needs to be observed to see if the atrial or ventricular rate is abnormal. Is the rate too fast or too slow for the patient's clinical condition? The atrial and ventricular rates also need to be examined to see if they are the same. The P:QRS ratio should be 1:1.

The QRS complex
The QRS complex should be examined to see if it is of the correct duration. The QRS should normally be less than 0.12 seconds. The complexes also need to be looked at to see if they are all the same and if they have a fixed relationship to the P wave. The P-R interval should also be measured.

Atrial activity
The atrial activity is assessed by examining the ECG to see if there are actual P waves or if there is a pattern of flutter or fibrillation. The P wave axis should be looked at to see if it is normal (normally 0 to 90 degrees) and the relationship between the P waves and the QRS complexes should be evaluated. The P waves should also be assessed to see if they all look alike.

Life-threatening arrhythmias are uncommon in children and are usually sinus in origin. Supportive interventions such as oxygen therapy can be as important as drug treatment for the arrhythmia. Arrhythmias can be categorized as either slow or fast.

Slow rhythms
Sinus bradycardia
This is a disorder of impulse formation. It is characterized by a pulse rate less than 100 in neonate, lower in an older child (McLeod 2003). The effects of sinus bradycardia are:

- increased preload
- decreased mean arterial pressure.

It is caused by:

- hypoxia
- hypokalaemia
- vagal stimulation.

Treatment involves:

- oxygen
- blood pressure support
- pacing.

Fast rhythms
Sinus tachycardia
The definition is dependent on the age of child but it is usually considered to be a rate 20 to 30 beats faster than normal. The effects of sinus tachycardia are:

- decreased filling time
- decreased MAP
- increased myocardial demand.

It is caused by:

- fever
- hypovolaemia
- stress, anxiety, pain
- early heart failure
- hypoxia.

Treatment involves:

- removing the underlying cause.

Supraventricular tachycardias
Supraventricular tachycardias (SVT) are the commonest arrhythmias of childhood and are the most common arrhythmia that produces cardiovascular instability during infancy (Wren 1999). SVT in infants usually produces a heart rate >220 bpm, and often 250–300 bpm. The QRS complex is narrow, making it difficult to differentiate between sinus tachycardia and SVT (Jones *et al.* 2005). SVT arise because the electrical conduction follows an abnormal pathway. The AV node often has dual pathways, an alpha and a beta pathway. In normal sinus rhythm the faster alpha pathway is used and accounts for the normal PR interval. When an SVT occurs the abnormal beta pathway is used and conduction differs from normal sinus rhythm. The diagnostic ECG feature of an SVT is that there are no P waves.
Acute treatment involves:

- Adenosine:
  - 50 μg/kg, 100 μg/kg, 250 μg/kg
  - rapid intravenous infusion
- Cardioversion:
  - 0.5 J/kg then 1–2 J/kg, synchronized shock
  - carotid sinus massage
  - Valsalva manoeuvre.

Ventricular tachycardia
Ventricular tachycardia consists of fast repeating ventricular beats. The complex is very wide on the ECG trace and P waves are absent. This arrhythmia severely compromises cardiac output. If the child is pulseless then it is treated in the same way as ventricular fibrillation, by defibrillation. If the child has a pulse then drugs are administered, usually lignocaine.

Ventricular fibrillation
There are no identifiable complexes on the ECG trace with this arrhythmia. It is rare in paediatrics and leads to no cardiac output.
   Causes:

- tricyclic antidepressants
- hypoxia
- hyperkalaemia.

The only useful treatment is resuscitation and defibrillation.

Case study 1: 4-day-old infant with suspected congenital cardiac disease

Leo is 4 days old and has been admitted to the High Dependency Unit from home. His mother noticed that he was very breathless when feeding and quite floppy. On admission his observations are:
   Respiratory rate 80 rpm, heart rate 160 bpm, temperature 37°C, oxygen saturation 85% in air. He looks centrally cyanosed and is peripherally cool. He also has some periorbital oedema.

Management
- What should your initial actions be?
  1. Complete ABC assessment.

2. Administer oxygen with caution as it is contraindicated in many types of congenital cardiac defect.
3. As Leo is centrally cyanosed he should be given no more than 30% oxygen until a diagnosis is made. If his condition worsens with the oxygen therapy it should be stopped.
- What monitoring does Leo require?
    1. Leo needs pulse oximetry and regular cardiovascular assessments to be undertaken including four-limb blood pressure.
    2. A diagnosis of TGA is made and arrangements are made to transfer Leo to the nearest cardiac unit for surgery.
- What medication should be administered?
    1. A prostaglandin infusion is started. Leo needs to be carefully monitored for side effects, particularly apnoea. He may need to be intubated for transfer if he has lots of apnoeic episodes.

Case study 2: 8-year-old with SVT

Stacey is 8 years old. She has a known diagnosis of SVT. She is admitted feeling unwell and complaining of palpitations. On admission her heart rate is unobtainable by feeling a pulse and the apex beat is too rapid to count.

Management

- What should your initial actions be?
    1. Complete ABC assessment.
    2. Attach cardiac monitor and 12-lead ECG.
- What manoeuvres should be attempted?
    1. Stacey could be encouraged to place her face in ice-cold water as this may help to terminate the SVT.
    2. Carotid sinus massage could also be attempted.
- What medication should be administered?
    1. Adenosine is the first drug of choice. Three incremental doses are given: 50 µg/kg, 100 µg/kg, 250 µg/kg.
    2. If adenosine is unsuccessful after three doses then cardioversion should be considered.

Conclusion

This chapter has explored assessment of a child with a cardiac disorder. It has also examined the different types of cardiac conditions that children may present within the HDU setting. Assessment and management of common arrhythmias has also been discussed. The nursing knowledge and interventions that have been covered in this chapter can also be used to inform the care of children who do not have an underlying cardiac problem but have suffered from cardiac failure due to another disease process.

 Learning activities

- Reflect upon the care of a child you have looked after who has an abnormal rhythm. What were the challenges of cardiac monitoring?
- Think about the impact a diagnosis of congenital cardiac disease has on a family. What do you think the long-term health implications might be? How would you help a family come to terms with this diagnosis?
- Reflect upon a child you have cared for with cardiac failure. What were the challenges presented by managing complex cardiac symptoms?

References and further reading

Archer N, Burch M (1998) *Paediatric Cardiology*. Chapman & Hall. London.

Cooke L, Steer P, Woodgate P (2003) Indomethacin for asymptomatic patent ductus arteriosus in preterm infants. *Cochrane Database of Systematic Reviews* Issue 1.

Davies MJ (2000) The cardiomyopathies: an overview. *Heart* **83**: 469–474.

Fleiner S (2006) Recognition and stabilization of neonates with congenital heart disease. *Newborn and Infant Nursing Reviews* **6**(3): 130–157.

Hia C, Yip W, Tai B, Quek S (2004) Immunosuppressive therapy in acute myocarditis: an 18-year systematic review. *Archives of Disease in Childhood* **89**: 580–584.

Horrox F (2002) *Manual of Neonatal and Paediatric Heart Disease*. Whurr Publishers Ltd, London.

Hudspeth R, O'Toole E (2000) Neonatal care: nursing care of neonates receiving intravenous prostaglandin E1 therapy who are not in an intensive care unit. *Critical Care Nurse* **20**(3): 62–68.

Jevon P, Ewens B (2007) *Monitoring the Critically Ill Patient*, 2nd Edition. Blackwell Publishing, Oxford.

Lee KJ, McCrindle BW, Bohn DJ *et al.* (1999) Clinical outcomes of acute myocarditis in childhood. *Heart* **82**(2): 226–233.

Leonard E (2004) Viral myocarditis. *Pediatric Infectious Disease Journal* **23**(7): 665–666.

Maconochie I (2004) Kawasaki Disease. *Archives of Disease in Childhood* **89** ep3–ep8.

McKenna W, Behr E (2002) Hypertrophic cardiomyopathy: management, risk stratification and prevention of sudden death. *Heart* **87**: 169–176.

McLeod K (2003) Syncope in childhood. *Archives of Disease in Childhood* **88**: 350–353.

Prendergast B (2004) Diagnostic criteria and problems in infective endocarditis. *Heart* **90**: 611–613.

Shaddy R (2001) Optimizing treatment for chronic congestive heart failure in children. *Critical Care Medicine* **29**(10 supp): 237–240.

Sheppard M, Wright M (2006) *Principles and Practice of High Dependency Nursing*. Bailliere Tindall, Edinburgh.

Sullivan B (2008) Nursing management of patients with a chest drain. *British Journal of Nursing* **17**(6): 388–393.

Westaby S, Franklin O, Burch M (1999) New developments in the treatment of cardiac failure. *Archives of Disease in Childhood* **81**: 276–277.

Westmoreland D (1999) Critical congenital cardiac defects in the newborn. *Journal of Perinatal and Neonatal Nursing* **12**(4): 67–87.

Williams C, Asquith J (2000) *Paediatric Intensive Care Nursing*. Churchill Livingstone, Edinburgh.

Wren C (1999) Catheter ablation in paediatric arrhythmias. *Archives of Disease in Childhood* **81**: 102–104.

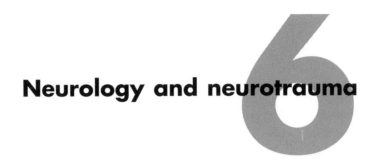

Neurology and neurotrauma

Helen Day and Andrea Cockett

Learning outcomes

- To develop an understanding of normal physiology and patho-physiology associated with intracranial pressure, cerebral blood flow and brain injury
- To develop an understanding of neurological assessment and investigations
- To develop an understanding of common neurological disorders such as infection and seizure activity

Introduction

The aim of this chapter is to provide the practitioner with the knowledge to care effectively for the child with neurological compromise. A frequently asked question in the hospital setting; 'Who should have neurological observation'? The answer is 'everyone'! It would clearly be inappropriate to perform a full set of neurological observations on all patients but it is paramount that all patients have their neurological status assessed. It must be remembered that the majority of patients in a high dependency unit are at risk of neurological deterioration or depression. There is pharmacology-related risk; for example, administration of morphine for postoperative analgesia or anticonvulsant medication may cause respiratory depression. Hypoxia-related neurological depression and cerebral oedema are risks for the general paediatric patient with respiratory distress. This chapter will address the specific complications of raised intracranial pressure, infection and seizure disorders.

Physiology

Neuro physiology is a vast and complex area. A understanding of the physiology of maintenance of cerebral perfusion and 'normal' intracranial pressure is required in the high dependency setting to allow recognition of neurological deterioration associated with infection, neurological disorder, trauma or surgery.

Cerebral circulation

Cerebral perfusion is the pressure gradient allowing blood flow to the brain (brain perfusion). It must be maintained within narrow limits because too little pressure could cause brain tissue to become ischaemic and too much could raise intracranial pressure (ICP).

CPP can be defined as the pressure gradient causing cerebral blood flow (CBF) such that:

$$CBF = CPP/CVR$$

where CVR is cerebrovascular resistance.

The three pressures that can contribute to the CPP are:

- mean arterial pressure (MAP)
- intracranial pressure (ICP)
- jugular venous pressure (JVP).

The cerebral circulation is unique in that there is a third pressure to consider in addition to venous and arterial pressures and this is the pressure external to the blood vessels; if this pressure is high it can restrict flow through the tissue. This situation is known as a Starling resistor. Such a situation exists in the brain where the external pressure is the ICP. Consequently, the correct definition of CPP is:

$$CPP = MAP - ICP \text{ (if ICP is higher than JVP, for example in serious head injury with brain swelling), or}$$

$$CPP = MAP - JVP \text{ (if JVP is higher than ICP).}$$

The pressure–volume relationship between ICP, volume of CSF, blood, and brain tissue, and cerebral perfusion pressure (CPP) is known as the Monro–Kellie doctrine or the Monro–Kellie hypothesis (Czos-nyka and Pickard 2003; Steiner and Andrews 2006; Duschek and Schandry 2007).

Intracranial pressure

Brain tissue and spinal fluid are relatively incompressible; the volume of the blood, the spinal fluid and brain in the cranium are relatively constant (Monro–Kellie doctrine). Therefore the cerebral vessels are compressed whenever the intracranial pressure rises. Any change in venous pressure promptly causes a similar change in intracranial pressure. Thus a rise in venous pressure decreases cerebral blood flow both by decreasing the effective perfusion pressure and by compressing the cerebral vessels. This relationship helps to compensate for changes in arterial blood pressure at the level of the head.

When ICP is elevated for more than a short period of time, CBF is significantly reduced. The resultant ischaemia stimulates the vasomotor area and systemic blood pressure rises, helping to maintain cerebral blood flow and perfusion pressure. Autoregulation is the process by which flow to many tissues is maintained at relatively constant levels despite variations in perfusion pressure. Autoregulation is prominent in the brain but can be compromised if there is significant brain swelling.

Data is limited describing normal values in infants and small children, however, under normal circumstances (MAP between 60 and 150 mmHg and ICP about 10 mmHg) cerebral blood flow is relatively constant due to protective autoregulation. Outside of the limits of autoregulation, raising MAP raises CPP and raising ICP lowers it, hence increasing ICP in traumatic brain injury is potentially deadly. CPP is normally between 70 and 90 mmHg in an adult human, and cannot be sustained below this level without risk of ischaemic brain damage, although some authorities regard 50–150 mmHg as a normal range for adults. Children require pressures of at least 60 mmHg.

One of the most damaging aspects of brain trauma and other conditions, directly correlated with poor outcome, is an elevated intracranial pressure. Very high intracranial pressures are often fatal if prolonged, but children can tolerate higher pressures for longer periods. An increase in pressure, most commonly due to head injury leading to intracranial haematoma or cerebral oedema can crush brain tissue, shift brain structures, contribute to hydrocephalus, cause the brain to herniate, and restrict blood supply to the brain, leading to an ischaemia and potential permanent damage to motor and cognitive function.

Causes of increased intracranial pressure

- *Mass/space occupying lesion* such as brain tumour, infarction with oedema, contusions, subdural or epidural haematoma, or abscess.
- *Generalized brain swelling* can occur in ischaemic-anoxia states, acute liver failure, hypertensive encephalopathy and hypercarbia.
- *Increase in venous pressure* can be due to venous sinus thrombosis, heart failure, or obstruction of superior mediastinal or jugular veins.
- *Obstruction to CSF flow and/or absorption* can occur in hydrocephalus (blockage in ventricles or subarachnoid space at base of brain, extensive meningeal disease (e.g. infectious, carcinomatous, granulomatous, or haemorrhagic).
- *Increased CSF production* can occur in meningitis, subarachnoid haemorrhage, or choroid plexus tumour.

Specific traumatic injuries

Pathology of brain injury

- *Contusion* represents a localized traumatic, necrotic and haemorrhagic lesion. Observed in approximately 40% of adults with sever traumatic brain injury (STBI) but less defined in children.
- *Haematoma* can be subdural, epidural or parenchymal. Incidence approximately 30% children under 4 years old and 17% in children aged 5–15.
- *Ischaemic injury* (neuronal necrosis and/or infarction) are common and key findings in STBI. They are seen in approximately 90% of fatal cases.
- *Axonal injury* is a unique finding in traumatic brain injury and can be local or diffuse. Stretching or transaction of axons by shearing forces is caused by a rotational acceleration -deceleration in injury. (Graham and Gennerali 2000; Ganong 2001)

Examination, observation and care of the neurological patient

It is evident from the causes of raised intracranial pressure listed above that many patients with the potential for raised intracranial pressure may be admitted to a high dependency unit; postoperative neurological surgery or children who have sustained a head injury. The word potential is vital in this specialty and early recognition of raised intracranial pressure or neurological depression is paramount in order to prevent permanent damage. Within the specialty of neurology and neurosurgery, specialist observations become the priority and it is difficult to apply the inspection, palpation and auscultation guide. However, always consider your respiratory and cardiovascular assessment findings when performing your neurological assessment as one system can have a profound effect on another.

AVPU as described in Chapter 2 is a useful rapid assessment tool but it is vital in a high dependency unit that a full neurological assessment can be performed. Level of consciousness is the first sign of deteriorating neurological status but the signs and symptoms are often missed or dismissed. Descriptive words such as irritability, drowsy and (dependent on age) incoherent, aggressive are misinterpreted as 'normal' or 'stress'. Compromised response and level of consciousness will be demonstrated in response to raised intracranial pressure considerably earlier than compromised vital signs and pupil responses. It is for this reason that the Glasgow coma score, the most widely used validated and prognostic score, focused on three areas of response: eye opening, verbal and motor (Teasdale and Jennett 1974) (Table 6.1).

The score for each indicator adds up to a total out of 15, with 15/15 being fully intact and 3/15 indicating imminent cardiorespiratory arrest and death. The score can further be broken down to indicate function with each component, for example E2 V2 M4 = GCS 8/15. It is now possible to see the comparative AVPU scores in more detail: A = GCS approximately 15/15, V = GCS approximately 11/15, P = GCS approximately 8/15 and U = GCS approximately 3/15.

Obviously smaller children will not be able to follow commands and have different motor responses, therefore an amended paediatric GCS is in common use (Table 6.2).

Table 6.1 Glasgow coma scale. Adapted from Teasdale and Jennett (1974).

Best eye response (E4)	No eye opening (1) Eye opening to pain (2) Eye opening to verbal command (3) Eyes open spontaneously (4)
Best verbal response (V5)	No verbal response (1) Incomprehensible sounds (2) Inappropriate words (3) Confused (4) Orientated (5)
Best motor response (M6)	No motor response (1) Extension to pain (2) Flexion to pain (3) Withdrawal from pain (4) Localizing pain (5) Obeys commands (6)

Table 6.2 Paediatric Glasgow coma scale. Adapted from Advanced Life Support Group (2007).

Best eye response (E4)	No eye opening (1)
	Eye opening to pain (2)
	Eye opening to verbal command (3)
	Eyes open spontaneously (4)
Best verbal response (V5)	No vocal response (1)
	Occasionally whimpers or moans (2)
	Cries inappropriately (3)
	Less than usual ability and/or spontaneous irritable cry (4)
	Alert, babbles, coos, words or sentences to usual ability (5)
Best motor response (M6)	No motor response to pain (1)
	Abnormal extension to pain (decerebrate) (arms) (2)
	Abnormal flexion to pain (decorticate) (arms) (3)
	Withdrawal from painful stimuli (4)
	Localizes to painful stimuli or withdraws to touch (5)
	Obeys commands or performs normal spontaneous movements (6)

Be aware that level of consciousness has two components:

1. Arousal (wakefulness); does the patient spontaneously or by stimulation of voice or pain open their eyes?
2. Awareness; questioning relating to orientation to person, place and time, or age-appropriate questions and distractions.

Failure to adequately stimulate the patient results in not being able to correctly identify their response. If your patient does not respond to voice at a level of shouting, then apply a painful stimulus. There is ongoing debate as to the best site. A sternal rub remains most practitioners' site of choice but there is an increasing change to using a trapezium squeeze as this is less traumatic for the patient. Pulling hair at the front hairline is becoming a popular choice in resuscitation teaching and may be more useful for smaller infants.

The motor response you wish to see is localizing to the point of pain … if the patient reaches for an intravenous line and starts tugging at it, this too is localizing, he just went to something else that irritated him! Peripheral pain stimulus may also be required (apply pressure to a pencil over the little moon on the cuticle) from patients who have not responded to a central stimulus or if everything moved apart from one limb.

Withdrawing is often misinterpreted; a simple reflex may be charted as withdrawing, but keep the stimulus going and if the patient continues to pull away then he is withdrawing. Posturing indicates serious injury. The two types are flexion (formerly decorticate) and extension (formerly decerebrate). In both postures the legs are rigidly extended.

Other early signs of raised intracranial pressure include nausea, vomiting and headache. Once you are satisfied with the level of consciousness and GCS, the remaining components of the neurological observations can be performed:

- Respiratory rate: Irregular respirations can occur dependent on the area of brain damaged. A slow respiratory rate is a particularly ominous sign and should be acted on immediately.
- Pulse: a widened pulse pressure and bradycardia are ominous signs. However, a tachycardia should not be ignored as it may be suggestive of shock that has not been adequately identified and treated.
- Blood pressure: elevated systolic blood pressure is a clinical sign of raised intracranial pressure and is often observed with a bradycardia. However do not discount other causes of hypertension if you are satisfied it is not associated with ICP, such as pain and anxiety.
- Function of cranial nerve III – pupil responses. Often referred to as a blown pupil, an increasing pupil size and decreased response to light is an ominous sign.

Bradycardia, hypertension and dilated pupils constitute what is known as Cushing's Triad and precede irreversible brain herniation.

The frequency of neurological observations will depend on the reason for admission to the high dependency unit. However, neurological deterioration can occur rapidly, and remember that the early signs of altered level of consciousness can easily be missed. Listen to the parents' description of their child's behaviour and perform full observations as indicated. Any patient recovering from a neurological or surgical event may be anxious and in pain. Ensure a quiet environment and effective use of appropriate age-related pain scores.

It is easy to focus on the neurological aspects of care at the expense other vital components of care. An elevated temperature increases cerebral metabolic demand, compromising a recovering brain. It may also be a sign of infection in the postoperative patient. Ensure your patient is prescribed antipyretics, monitor the effect and act on signs of infection; send blood cultures and wound swabs and ensure wound dressings are clean and dry and drains intact.

Report any drop in GCS as a matter of urgency to the medical team and ensure that emergency equipment is at hand.

Investigations

There are some specific investigations that can facilitate optimum care and potential need for intervention. However these specialist investigations invariably mean transferring the child around the hospital. A multidisciplinary decision must be made, taking into account the benefits versus the potential risk of transfer, such as unnecessary noise, trauma and movement. If the child does need to be moved to another department ensure that you have the necessary equipment with you to resuscitate and maintain airway, breathing and circulation, and consider calling in expert assistance if sedation is required. Occasionally a lumbar puncture may be performed in order to analyse the cerebrospinal fluid for signs of infection or haemorrhage. There is evidence to suggest that a lumbar puncture is contraindicated where raised ICP is suspected and expert advice should be sought. There are many specialist investigations beyond the scope of this book but the most commonly available are listed below:

1. *Computed tomography scan:* series of cross-sectional (axial) images. Can be classified as invasive as contrast dyes may be injected.
2. *Magnetic resonance imaging:* non-invasive, non-radiation exposure used to delineate tumours, oedema, ischaemic and haemorrhagic lesions, hydrocephalus, vascular disorders, inflammatory and infectious lesions and degenerative processes.
3. *Electroencephalogram:* non-invasive electrophysiological method for recording cerebral activity, has its greatest application in the study of seizure disorders.
4. *Cerebrospinal fluid sampling:* normal pressure 50–150 mmH$_2$O, normal colour is colourless.

Management of head injury

Young children are at greater risk of head injury due to the higher ratio of the head size in relation to the rest of the body. Mechanism of head injury varies with age. Road traffic accidents are the commonest cause of head injury in school-age children. Infants and preschool children usually sustain injuries from falls and non-accidental injury. Children presenting with head injury need swift treatment if further morbidity is to be avoided. Any child who presents to hospital with a GCS of less than 8 should be intubated and transfer arranged to a PICU. Any child whose GCS deteriorates while on the high dependency unit will also need to be intubated and transferred to the appropriate clinical area. Immediate priorities when a child with a head injury is admitted are:

- ABC assessment
- Glasgow coma score
- Pain relief as pain has been shown to increase the intracranial pressure
- Urgent referral for CT scan within 1 hour if any of the following conditions are met:
  - Loss of consciousness lasting more than 5 minutes (witnessed)
  - Amnesia lasting more than 5 minutes
  - Abnormal drowsiness
  - Three or more discrete episodes of vomiting
  - Clinical suspicion of non-accidental injury
  - Post-traumatic seizure with no history of epilepsy
  - For an infant GCS less than 14, for a child GCS less than 15
  - Suspicion of an open or closed skull fracture or a tense fontanelle
  - Any sign of a basal skull fracture
  - Focal neurological deficit
  - If under 1 year, presence of bruising, swelling or laceration more than 5 cm on the head
  - Dangerous mechanism of injury (high speed crash, fall greater than 3 m, high speed collision or impact with an object) (National Institute for Clinical Excellence 2007).

If non-accidental injury is suspected then a clinician with experience of safeguarding procedures will need to be involved in the immediate and ongoing care of the child. This may require a full body survey to be undertaken to check for other injuries. It is important that only a limited number of clinicians are involved in taking the history to ensure that information is correctly documented.

Types of head injury

Scalp injuries can either be abrasions, which are breaks in the top layer of the skin, or lacerations, which are tears in the scalp tissues. Lacerations can bleed excessively and a record of blood loss may need to be made.

Skull fractures are dependent upon the speed, direction and momentum of the causative impact. Linear fractures are the most common seen in children. The bone remains in alignment and the dura is not damaged. Comminuted fractures result from fragmentation of the bone or multiple fracture lines. Depressed skull fractures are characterized by an inward depression of skull fragments. The dura remains intact. Basal skull fractures involve damage to the dura resulting in leakage of CSF. Haemorrhage can also occur with a basal skull fracture.

Brain injury is characterized as either being diffuse or focal. Diffuse injuries include contusion, which is bruising to the brain. Hypoxic-ischaemic injury is caused by impaired cerebral perfusion following a head injury and diffuse axonal injury is caused by the forces of acceleration/deceleration that occur during head trauma. Focal brain injuries are usually contusions and lacerations that occur either at the site of impact or on the opposite side of the brain to the impact.

Haemorrhage can occur in children. It is classified as either extradural or intradural. Extradural haemorrhage is normally associated with fracture of the temporal bone. The middle meningeal artery is damaged, causing a rapid haematoma. This requires immediate surgical intervention. Intradural haemorrhages are usually a combination of subdural and intracerebral haematomas. These are slow to grow and can usually be managed medically.

Secondary brain damage can occur following the initial injury. It is usually caused by a combination of factors including hypercapnia, hypoxia, infection, ischaemia and raised intracranial pressure.

Neurological observations need to be carried out frequently for the first 6 hours following head injury. This is because these initial hours have been identified as the time in which a deterioration or complications are most likely to occur (NICE 2007). Following initial assessment within the emergency department, observations should be carried out:

- half-hourly for the first 2 hours
- hourly for the next 4 hours
- 2 hourly from this point onwards (NICE 2007).

This regime only applies to patients who have a GCS of 15. If the GCS is less than 15 or the GCS drops below 15 during the observation period then the observations will need to be undertaken more frequently. Other factors that need to be taken into consideration when deciding frequency of observations include the patient becoming more agitated or exhibiting abnormal behaviour, vomiting, headache, abnormal movements or pupil changes. Any of these clinical indicators should lead to reassessment by a doctor and increase in the frequency of observations.

Nursing interventions for head injury

Management of head injury patients is primarily focused on observing their condition for deterioration and surgical intervention if required. There are some nursing interventions that should be utilized when caring for this group of patients. These interventions are aimed at reducing the risk of raised intracranial pressure and they include:

- providing oxygen therapy if required to increase cerebral oxygenation;
- nursing the child in an upright position (30° tilt) with the head in the midline;
- fluid balance monitoring;
- minimal handling;
- effective pain management.

Infectious disorders

Table 6.3 lists some of the infectious causes of neurological disorder.

Meningitis

Meningitis is a systemic disease that primarily affects the meninges of the brain. It can be bacterial or viral. Outbreaks occur every 10 to 15 years and these can be clustered in geographical locations. It is more

Table 6.3 Infectious disorders and causative organisms.

Disease	Infective organism
Viral meningitis	Echo virus Coxsackie virus Chickenpox (varicella-zoster virus) Herpes virus Polio virus Mumps (paramyxovirus)
Bacterial meningitis	Meningococcus Pneumococcus Hib (*Haemophilus influenzae* type B)
TB meningitis	*Mycobacterium tuberculosis*
Listeriosis	*Listeria monocytogenes* Gram-positive bacteria
Neonatal meningitis	*E. coli* Group B streptococci

common in children under 5, teenagers and young people (Wong 2001). Children under 1 are the most commonly affected group and mortality is also highest in this group. Morbidity following meningitis can be high and children may suffer hearing loss and more seriously mental and physical disability following infection.

Bacterial meningitis usually involves infection of the pia and arachnoid space. Causative organisms enter the body via the upper respiratory tract and then reach the subarachnoid space and meninges indirectly through the nasal mucosa from where they enter the bloodstream. The presence of the bacteria leads to brain congestion, oedema and ischaemia. This presents itself as raised intracranial pressure.

Signs and symptoms

Meningitis manifests as a flu-like illness with early signs of pyrexia, vomiting and malaise. Specific symptoms include:

- severe headache;
- stiff neck;
- drowsiness;
- photophobia;
- joint pain;
- poor feeding;
- irritability;
- high-pitched cry;
- seizures;
- positive Kernig sign (pain associated with the flexion of the upper leg and then extension of the knee);
- positive Brudzinski sign (flexion of the knees and hips in response to flexion of the head and neck);
- petechial rash is associated with meningococcal disease.

Diagnosis of meningitis is usually made from CSF examination following lumbar puncture. Lumbar puncture however should not be attempted in children with raised intracranial pressure. In this situation the child should be treated for the most common causative agent.

Management of meningitis involves admission to hospital, isolation, antibiotic therapy if it is bacterial, fluid management and symptomatic treatment of pain and fever. Nursing interventions required include:

- temperature assessment and antipyretic measures
- administration of antibiotics
- neurological assessment
- pain assessment and management
- seizure monitoring and management
- awareness of the potential for raised intracranial pressure.

Encephalitis

Encephalitis is an acute inflammation of the brain and occasionally the meninges (Slota 1998). It occurs more frequently in children under the age of 10 and is more common in children who are immunosuppressed (Wong 2001). It is usually viral in origin.

Signs and symptoms
The signs and symptoms of encephalitis can vary widely depending upon the severity of the infection. Flu-like illness is usually a precursor and specific symptoms include:

- malaise
- upper respiratory tract symptoms
- nausea
- vomiting
- neck stiffness.

Deterioration manifests itself through:

- lethargy
- drowsiness
- coma
- seizures
- symptoms of raised intracranial pressure.

Management of encephalitis is similar to meningitis but because it is usually viral in origin only supportive measures are usually useful.

Seizures

Seizures are brief malfunctions of the brain's electrical system resulting from cortical neuronal discharge. The manifestations of seizures are determined by the site of origin and may include unconsciousness or altered consciousness, involuntary movements, and changes in perception, behaviours, sensations and postures (Wong 2001).

Causes of seizures

It is important to establish the reason for a seizure so that the appropriate intervention can be identified. A number of conditions can lead to seizures:

- Epilepsy
- Infections either systemic (febrile convulsion) or neurological (meningitis, encephalitis)

- Abscess
- Head injury
- Structural lesions, space-occupying lesion, tumour
- Cerebral infarction, haematoma, intraventricular haemorrhage (IVH)
- Hypoxia
- Acidosis
- Metabolic disorders
- Electrolyte imbalances: hypocalcaemia, hypoglycaemia, hyponatraemia, hypernatraemia, dehydration
- Toxic ingestion
- Hypoxic ischaemic encephalopathy (HIE).

Types of seizure

Focal seizures which start in a part or focus of the brain include focal sensory seizures, focal motor seizures and secondary generalized seizures.

Generalized seizures include absence, myoclonic, clonic, tonic-clonic, tonic and atonic seizures.

Focal seizures
Focal sensory seizures
There are a great variety of focal sensory siezures; they usually assume the same form in one person and it is unusual for them to occur alone. Children often go on to develop another form of partial seizure. Consciousness and normal awareness are maintained during the seizure.

Manifestations include:

- twitching of a limb
- pins and needles
- rising feeling in the stomach
- unusual taste
- some sensory disturbance
- feelings of *'deja-vu'* or fear.

Focal motor seizures
There is an alteration in consciousness with focal motor seizures and they usually present as altered or automatic behaviour. They can develop from simple seizures.

Manifestations include:

- lip smacking or chewing movements
- plucking at clothing, fiddling with objects
- acting in a confused manner

- grimacing, undressing
- performing semi-purposive movements
- walking around in a drunken fashion.

Secondary generalized seizures
These are partial seizures, either simple or complex, in which discharge spreads to the whole brain. This can happen so rapidly that only an EEG can show that the seizure originated in one area. This type of seizure has the same characteristics as a generalized tonic-clonic seizure.

Generalized seizures
Generalized seizures start all over the brain and there are six groups.

Absence seizures (petit mal)

- There is a brief interruption of consciousness during which blank staring, fluttering of eyelids and head nodding may occur.
- Duration is only a few seconds and it may go unnoticed.

Atonic seizures

- Onset and cessation is not as abrupt as an absence seizure.
- Can cause akinetic drop attacks, where the child drops to the floor with such force they need to wear a crash helmet.

Myoclonic seizures

- Typified by abrupt, brief, shock-like jerks.
- These may involve the whole body, arms or head.
- Often occur shortly after waking.
- The child may fall but recovery is immediate.

Clonic seizures

- Similar to tonic-clonic without the tonic component.

Tonic seizures

- Sudden stiffening of muscles.
- Child becomes rigid and falls.
- There is no jerking.
- Usually quick recovery.
- Convulsions stop after about 5 minutes.

Tonic-clonic seizures (grand mal)

- Tonic phase starts with a sudden explosion of air.
- This results in a high-pitched cry.
- Child becomes rigid, falls to the ground and shakes all over.
- Breathing is laboured and there is cyanosis and excessive salivation.
- Incontinence can occur.
- Convulsions stop after about 5 minutes.
- After the convulsions there is deep respiration and the child regains consciousness but may be confused.

The nursing care required for a child having a seizure is the same irrespective of the type or cause of the seizure. A seizure lasting for more than a few minutes must be treated. The sustained seizure activity increases the adenosine triphosphate (ATP) requirements of neurons, as the constant electrical activity requires an extremely active sodium-potassium pump. Systemic physiological changes occur early in a seizure. These changes include increased cerebral blood flow with increase in oxygen and glucose delivery to the brain and increased removal of toxic metabolites. Heart rate and blood pressure increase as do blood glucose levels. Respiratory function can be compromised in some seizures and this leads to decreased oxygenation. After about 30 minutes these physiological mechanisms fail and probably contribute to any neurological damage that may occur. Eventually this can lead to hypoxaemia or apnoea and hypoglycaemia caused by the increased metabolic activity in skeletal muscles (Hazinski 1992). As a result cellular exhaustion and selected cellular destruction can occur.

Common conditions

Febrile convulsions

Febrile convulsions occur in 3 to 4% of children under 5 years (Miller 1996). They are brief and self limiting. The peak incidence for occurrence is 6 months to 3 years (Wong 2001). Their pathogenesis is unknown but a familial incidence indicates a genetic predisposition to febrile convulsions.

Clinical characteristics:

- Rare before 6 months and after 5 years.
- The convulsion occurs with a rise in temperature to >38 °C.
- Usually occurs with upper respiratory tract infections or otitis media.
- Most seizures occur within the first 24 hours of the illness.

- The seizure is short (less than 15 minutes), generalized and predominately tonic.
- Interictal EEG is normal.
- The seizure does not normally reoccur in the same illness.
- No acute systemic metabolic disorder is present.

Factors that contribute to susceptibility include age, degree and rate of temperature elevation and the nature of the fever inducing illness. Some children develop complex febrile seizures which have a duration of more than 15 minutes, they have focal characteristics, they usually occur more than once in a 24-hour period and they are considered a risk factor for developing epilepsy (Miller 1996).

Epilepsy

Repeated recurrence of seizure activity is known as epilepsy. Over 75% of individuals with epilepsy start to have seizures before they reach 18 years of age. Approx 100,000 children and young people have epilepsy in the UK (Buelow 2001). The disorganized electrical activity that takes place in epilepsy does not lead to neuronal death but can result in damage to delicate areas of the brain such as the hippocampus if the seizures are long and frequent. This can lead to the development of other epileptic foci. Status epilepticus can lead to brain anoxia.

Nursing interventions for a child with seizures

Management of a child with seizures requires the maintenance of vital functions, abolition of seizures, elimination of any precipitating factors and reversing of correctable causes. One of the most important aspects of managing seizures in children is detailed documentation. Accurate recording of the duration and nature of a seizure is very important both in children who have a known condition and those for whom it is their first seizure.

With all children the first principle to observe is that of ABC:

- Maintenance of a patent airway.
- Assessment and support of breathing.
- Assessment and support of circulation.

Working oxygen and suction should be to hand, as should an appropriately sized bag mask valve device. The child should be nursed on their side and efforts should be made to ensure the environment is safe. The seizure should be timed and any manifestations should be noted. Prescribed medication should be administered and its effectiveness noted. If the seizure does not respond then a further dose of medication can be administered. The child should never be left unattended and help should be summoned (Buelow 2001).

Status epilepticus

Status epilepticus is a medical emergency. It is defined as 'any seizure lasting for a duration of at least 30 minutes or repeated seizures lasting for 30 minutes or longer from which the patient does not regain consciousness' (Appleton 1998). Management of status epilepticus (Fig. 6.1) adheres to the same principles as management of any other seizure, with ABC being the priority. Oxygen is usually administered and observations need to be carefully monitored. Intravenous anticonvulsant medication is usually required. If the seizure is very prolonged then the child may require intubation and ventilation.

Management

- What should be your initial actions?
  1. Complete a GCS assessment; if GCS is still 15 perform a full assessment of all systems to provide a comprehensive baseline condition.
  2. Explain to Simon and his parents what you are doing and the reasons why.
- Does Simon need additional monitoring and oxygen therapy?
  1. An oxygen saturation monitor and an automated blood pressure machine will be helpful adjuncts but not essential as your own assessment of GCS will be most useful.
  2. Oxygen therapy should not be required. The development of an oxygen requirement should alert you to deterioration in clinical condition.
- How often should you perform neurological observations?
  1. Every 30 minutes initially: skulls are hard but so is concrete and he fell 3 metres. Always consider the mode of injury when planning your care. Remember the important 'P' word – potential.
  2. Utilize your early warning scoring system, if in place, with your observations.
- What else may Simon need?
  1. Simon is feeling sick which is common after a bang to the head. If Simon cannot tolerate sips of water he may need some intravenous fluids. There is no need to restrict fluids in the high dependency setting for uncomplicated head injuries; hydration and normal blood pressure are required for brain and tissue perfusion.
- Consider:
  1. Potential for deterioration associated with mode of injury.
  2. Preparation for transfer to CT or MRI scan if GCS decreases.

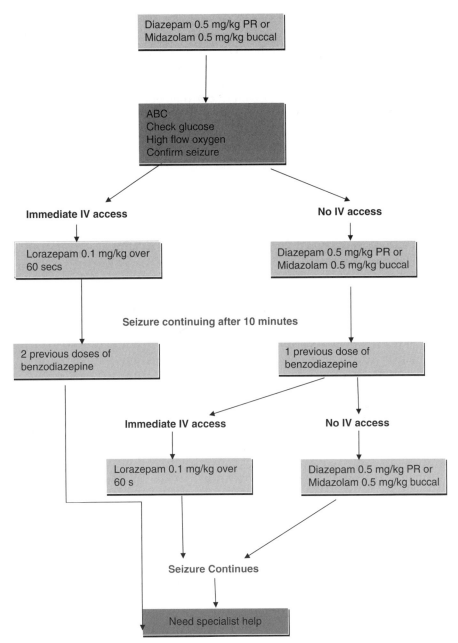

Figure 6.1 Pathway for the management of status epilepticus. Adapted from British Paediatric Neurology Association (2004).

3. A useful drug to have with your emergency equipment is mannitol. In the intensive care setting there are alternatives but mannitol is conveniently available ready to administer. Mannitol is an osmotic diuretic that is effective for control of raised ICP. Effective doses range from 0.25/kg to 1g/kg. Mannitol should be only be given under the supervision of a consultant intensivist or anaesthetist.

4. Inform outreach team, intensive care or senior staff that you have Simon, so you have help at hand should you need it.

Case study 1: 6-year-old with acute head injury

Simon, a 6-year-old boy, has been admitted to the high dependency unit after sustaining a head injury caused by falling approximately 3 metres from a climbing frame onto concrete. He was not knocked out but paramedics report his GCS to have been 13/15 on their arrival at the scene. His GCS on admission is 15/15 but he complains of feeling sick. He has a bruise on the left side of his forehead. No CT scan was performed and emergency department staff removed his cervical spine collar when they were satisfied that he had no neck injury.

Case study 2: 3-year-old suffering from a seizure

Sarah, a 3-year-old girl, has been admitted following a seizure. She has had one seizure in the emergency department and is transferred to the high dependency unit. The seizure in the emergency department lasted 3 minutes. She has no fever and no history of a preceding illness or trauma. Her mother has noticed that for the past few weeks she has periods in the day where she appears to be daydreaming and does not respond when her mother calls her.

Management

- What should your initial actions be?
  1. Complete ABC assessment.
  2. Ensure oxygen and suction are available and working.
  3. Complete a GCS assessment.
- What monitoring does Sarah require?
  1. Sarah needs pulse oximetry and regular neurological and cardiovascular assessments to be undertaken.
- Does Sarah require oxygen therapy?
  1. If Sarah has another seizure and it lasts longer than 5 minutes then high flow oxygen should be started.
- Sarah starts to fit again; what observations do you need to take?
  1. You need to note the time of the start of the seizure and look for any movements involved, this should all be recorded on a seizure chart.
  2. Sarah should be placed on her side.
  3. You need to observe her oxygen saturation levels.
- What medication should be administered?
  1. Diazepam 0.5 mg/kg rectally or midazolam 0.5 mg/kg buccally can be administered.
  2. Paraldehyde can also be administered rectally.
- What would you do if the seizure does not stop?
  1. Specialist help with diagnosis and management needs to be sought form a neurological consultant.
  2. Sarah may need to be transferred to a PICU for seizure management.
- Sarah's family are very anxious.
  1. Sarah and her family will need lots of support during this time, there may be a specialist epilepsy nurse in the area who can help them understand the diagnosis and the management required.

Conclusion

This chapter has discussed the anatomy and physiology of the neurological system and identified some common conditions that you may encounter in the high dependency setting. Nursing interventions for managing these conditions have been identified and also the current guidance about treatment.

Learning activities

- Review the principles of neurological assessment and consider how the early signs of neurological deterioration may be missed in young children.
- Write a care plan for a 7-year-old who has fallen off his bike, has probably had no loss of consciousness but the accident was not witnessed has been admitted for observation as he has vomited twice.
- Formulate a discussion on the benefits of a vaccination programme that protects against meningococcal meningitis. Consider cost and clinical outcomes.
- Consider the stigma that a child who suffers from epilepsy may encounter and what education could be provided to schools in order to prevent this.

References and further reading

Advanced Life Support Group (2007) *Advanced Paediatric Life Support: the practical approach*. Blackwell Publishing, Oxford.

Appleton R, Gibbs J (1998) *Epilepsy in Childhood and Adolescence*, 2nd Edition. Martin Dunitz, London.

British Paediatric Neurology Association (2004) Convulsive Status Epilepticus. bpna.org.uk/audit/Status%20epilepticus.pdf. BPNA (accessed: 21 July 2008).

Buelow J (2001) Epilepsy management issues and techniques. *Journal of Neuroscience Nursing* **33**(5): 260–269.

Duschek S, Schandry R (2007) Reduced brain perfusion and cognitive performance due to constitutional hypotension. *Clinical Autonomic Research* **17**(2): 69–76.

Czosnyka M, Pickard JD (2004) Monitoring and interpretation of intracranial pressure. *Journal of Neurology, Neurosurgery, and Psychiatry* **75**(6): 813–821.

Ganong W (2001) *Review of Medical Physiology*, 21st Edition. Lange Medical, New York.

Graham DI, Gennareli TA (2000) Pathology of brain damage after head injury. In Cooper P, Golfinos G (eds) *Head Injury*, 4th Edition. Morgan Hill, New York.

Hazinski M (1992) *Nursing Care of the Critically Ill Child*, 2nd Edition. Mosby-Year Book Inc, St Louis, MO.

Lower J (2002) Facing neuro assessment fearlessly. *Nursing* **32**(2): 58–65.

Miller R (1996) The effect on parents of febrile convulsions. *Paediatric Nursing* **8**(9): 28–31.

National Institute for Clinical Excellence (2007) *Head Injury Triage: assessment, investigation and early management of head injury in infants, children and adults.* NICE, London.

Slota M (1998) *Core Curriculum for Pediatric Critical Care Nursing.* WB Saunders, Philadelphia.

Steiner LA, Andrews PJ (2006) Monitoring the injured brain: ICP and CBF. *British Journal of Anaesthesia* **97**(1): 26–38.

Teasdale G, Jennett B (1974) Assessment of coma and impaired consciousness: A practical scale. *Lancet* **2**: 81–84.

Wong D (2001) *Wong's Essentials of Pediatric Nursing,* 6th Edition. Mosby Inc, St Louis, MO.

Gastrointestinal and renal systems

Leanne Burns and Andrea Cockett

Learning outcomes

- To develop an understanding of the normal anatomy and physiology of the gastrointestinal and renal systems
- To develop an understanding of abdominal examination and nutrition in relation to high-dependency care assessment and investigations
- To develop an understanding of gastrointestinal and renal conditions that may be encountered in the high dependency setting

Introduction

The aim of this chapter is to discuss the anatomy and physiology of both the gastrointestinal and renal systems. Assessment of each system will be covered and common conditions and their management discussed.

Gastrointestinal system

Anatomy and physiology

The gastrointestinal (GI) system consists of all organs that are concerned in the chewing, swallowing, digestion and absorption of food as well as the elimination of indigestible and undigested foods (Watson 2005). The gastrointestinal system comprises two major divisions, the gastrointestinal tract and the accessory organs (Waugh and Grant 2006, Wolters Kluwer Health 2008).

The various parts making up this tract are:

- *Mouth* – primarily the tongue and teeth. Digestive processes begin here with chewing, salivating and swallowing (Waugh and Grant 2006).
- *Pharynx* – allows the passage of food from the mouth to the oesophagus. The epiglottis is located directly behind the roof of the tongue and closes to protect the larynx when food is being swallowed.
- *Oesophagus* – moves food from the pharynx to the stomach. As food is swallowed the upper oesophageal sphincter relaxes, food moves into the oesophagus, with peristalsis then assisting in food moving to the stomach (Kindlen 2003, Smith and Watson 2005).
- *Stomach* – lies in the left upper abdominal quadrant. Contains two sphincters: the cardiac sphincter protecting the entrance to the stomach and the pyloric sphincter guarding the exit. Functions of the stomach include temporary storage of food, mixing of food with gastric juices to liquefy contents to chyme, movement of chyme into the small intestine, secretion of gastrin (hormone) and production and secretion of intrinsic factor needed for absorption of vitamin B12 (Patton 2006).
- *Small intestine* – comprises the duodenum, the jejunum and the ileum or terminal section ending at the ileocaecal valve. The absorption of proteins, carbohydrates and fats takes place through the villi in the small intestine. Peristalsis promotes the movement of chyme through the small intestine where it mixes with enzymes from the pancreas, bile from the liver and hormones aiding digestion (Weber and Kelley 2006).
- *Large intestine* – also known as the colon. Extends from the end of the ileum to the anus. Divided into seven sections known: as the caecum; ascending, transverse, descending and sigmoid colons; the rectum and the anus (Watson 2005). Functions include absorbing water and electrolytes, storage of food residue and elimination of waste in the form of faeces. A summary of gastrointestinal tract functions can be seen in Table 7.1.

The accessory organs of the gastrointestinal system include the liver, pancreas, gallbladder and bile ducts.

- *Liver* – located in the right upper quadrant of the abdomen underneath the diaphragm. Has two major lobes divided by the falciform ligament. The liver is unique in that it has a dual blood supply. The

Table 7.1 Summary of GI tract function. Adapted from Long (2002).

Function	Mechanism involved	Where it occurs
Digestion of food	Mastication Swallowing Enzymatic digestion Absorption	Mouth (teeth and tongue) Oropharynx Stomach, small intestine Stomach, small and large intestine
Motility	Peristalsis, mass movement	Throughout gut
Storage of food waste		Stomach, sigmoid colon, rectum
Excretion	Defecation	Rectum and anus
Endocrine secretions	Gastrin secretion Secretin secretion Insulin secretion	Stomach Duodenal mucosa Pancreas
Defence	Smell, sight, taste Gastric and secretion Vomit reflex Gut flora, mucus secretion Immune response	Oral cavity, cephalic region Stomach Stomach up to mouth Throughout gut Peyer's patches (aggregations of lymphoid tissue present in gut walls), macrophages in mucosa

hepatic artery carrying oxygen-rich blood contributes about 25% of the blood supply. The portal vein delivers the rest. The portal vein carries blood rich in nutrients and metabolic by-products of digestion from the gastrointestinal tract. Blood exits the liver through the hepatic vein and into the inferior vena cava (IVC) (Whiteman and McCormick 2005). Functions of the liver include: metabolism of fat and glucose; synthesis and storage of glycogen; breakdown of amino acids to form urea; synthesis of proteins (including clotting factors and albumin); breakdown of drugs and toxins; storage of soluble vitamins A, D, E and K, activation of vitamin D, storage of water-soluble vitamins e.g. vitamin B12, glycogen (converted from glucose under the influence of insulin), iron (from diet and red blood cells) and copper; phagocytosis of worn-out red and white blood cells as well as some bacteria; production of bile – formed from constituents brought by blood. Bile is composed of water, bile salts, cholesterol and bile pigments (mainly bilirubin). Primary functions of bile are to emulsify and saponify fats; aid cholesterol and fatty acids to become soluble, ensuring these and fat soluble vitamins (A, D, E and K) can be absorbed, transportation of bilirubin ready for conversion to an excretable form, and deodorization of faeces.

- *Pancreas* – lies horizontally in the abdomen behind the stomach. Structurally it can be divided into three regions; the head which lies over the vena cava in the curve of the duodenum, the body which lies behind the duodenum, and the tail which is situated under the spleen (Smith and Watson 2005; Watson 2005). The pancreas is an exocrine and endocrine gland. The function of the exocrine pancreas is to produce pancreatic juice containing enzymes assisting in digestion of fats, proteins and carbohydrates (Waugh and Grant 2006). The endocrine pancreas secretes insulin and glucose directly into the blood. The most common endocrine disorder in childhood is type 1 diabetes mellitus (T1DM) affecting about 2% of the population. This is an autoimmune disease arising when a child with a predisposition is exposed to a precipitating event (usually a viral infection). Islet cells present in the pancreas responsible for the production of insulin are particularly susceptible to viral damage and, should this occur, a decrease in effective circulating insulin prevails. Insulin is a hormone acting to lower blood glucose levels in several ways including accelerating the transport of glucose from blood into cells, increasing the rate of glucose conversion into glycogen (glycogenesis), decreasing glycogenolysis and gluconeogenesis and accelerating the transport of amino acids from blood into cells. When islet cells are damaged, insulin deficiency accelerates the breakdown of the body's fat reserves, resulting in the production of ketones (organic acids). Catabolism of stored fats and proteins occurs to ensure a constant energy supply to the body, resulting in weight loss, polyuria and excessive thirst.

- *Gall bladder* – a pear-shaped sac attached to the posterior surface of the liver. Its primary function is to concentrate, store and release bile (Long 2002; Waugh and Grant 2006).
- *Bile ducts* – the hepatic and cystic ducts merge to form the common bile duct which passes down behind the head of the pancreas. Bile produced in the liver travels into the hepatic duct, then the cystic duct and into the gall bladder where it is concentrated, stored and released as required. Once released, bile moves through the common bile duct and into the duodenum where it assists in processes of digestion.

Now that a review of the components of the gastrointestinal tact has been undertaken, focus will be directed towards the assessment of this tract and accessory organs. Throughout, common paediatric anomalies will be highlighted and assessment findings related to these anomalies discussed.

Clinical assessment

For the purpose of assessment the abdomen is divided into four quadrants by imaginary vertical and horizontal lines bisecting the umbilicus.

Table 7.2 Summary of quadrant contents.

Quadrant	Composition
Right upper	Right lobe of liver, gall bladder, pylorus, duodenum, head of pancreas, hepatic flexure of colon, portions of the ascending and transverse colon
Left upper	Left lobe of liver, stomach, body of pancreas, splenic flexure of colon, portions of the transverse and descending colon
Right lower	Cecum and appendix, portion of the ascending colon
Left lower	Sigmoid colon, portion of the descending colon

These quadrants are known as the right upper quadrant, left upper quadrant, right lower quadrant and left lower quadrant. The organs within each quadrant are detailed in Table 7.2.

History

History taking is key to determining abdominal pathophysiology in association with the abdomen. History should be taken from both the child (age dependent) and parent. Particular focus should be directed towards obtaining information about previous abdominal problems, changes in behaviour (fatigue, mood swings), changes in appetite, difficulty in swallowing, food intolerances, abdominal pain, nausea/vomiting, bowel habits and current medications, with an overview of nutritional intake gained. A good history can provide clues to the aetiology of the underlying problems. Following the history taking, examination continues with inspection. Explanation of the procedures should be given to the child and family at all times.

Inspection

Abdominal assessment begins, as all other systems assessment, with inspection. Inspection of nfants and toddlers can be challenging; asking the parent to place the infant on their knee can be more conducive to a thorough assessment. If possible lay the child on a bed and stand at their right side.

- Contour: Stoop and gaze across the abdomen to determine the profile from the rib margin to the pubic bone. This is normally flat and rounded (Jarvis 2004). The abdomen in toddlers and children is usually protuberant in the upright position and it can be difficult to distinguish a normal 'pot belly' from a pathological one (Gill and O'Brien. 2004). Abdominal distension is often gaseous but further assessment will help determine whether distention is from fat, fluid, faeces, flatus or visceromegaly. Visible loops of bowel may be noted in malnourished infants.

- Symmetry: Shining a light across the abdomen will demonstrate whether symmetry is present. Particular attention should be given to any localized bulging, visible masses or asymmetry. In male infants common findings include inguinal hernias. Wilms' tumours can come to attention when parents describe noting a swelling when bathing their child.
- Umbilicus: The umbilicus should be midline and inverted with no sign of discoloration, inflammation or hernia. Children with liver disease and ascites may present with an everted umbilicus. The presence of an umbilical hernia will also result in an everted umbilicus. This can also be evident with an underlying mass.
- Skin: Note the skin surface. It should be smooth and even with homogenous colour. Skin that appears taut may indicate underlying ascites. Ascities occurs with liver disease when production of albumin and clotting factors diminishes, reducing plasma osmotic pressure, resulting in a movement of fluid into interstitial space, eventually resulting in accumulation in the peritoneal cavity. A yellow discoloration of the skin is indicative of jaundice caused by deposits of bile pigments due to a disruption of the flow of bile through the common bile ducts or hepatic ducts (Smith and Watson 2005). The appearance of spider-like veins across the abdomen underneath the skin is suggestive of portal hypertension (increased pressure within the portal system as a result of liver disease causing the development of collateral circulation to and around the liver to assist with pressure reduction) (Whiteman and McCormick 2005). Check and document any operative scars you may inspect. The presence of lesions and rashes should also be noted. Childhood diseases such as measles and chicken pox can result in rashes across the abdomen.
- Pulsation/Movement – Respiration is usually abdominal in children until they reach school age. Pulsations from the aorta may be observed in the epigastric region in thin children. Marked visible peristalsis in conjunction with a distended abdomen indicates intestinal obstruction. Intussusception is the most frequent cause of intestinal obstruction in the first two years of life (Sondheimer 2004). On inspection a distended abdomen is generally noted and the infant or toddler is often screaming and drawing up their knees.

While utilizing skills of inspection is it also important to observe the child's behaviour. Are they still and quiet? Are they restless and unable to find a comfortable position? Observe facial features as this can provide evidence of the severity of pain experienced by the child.

Auscultation

Auscultation is usefully performed before percussion and palpation when conducting an abdominal assessment, as these may increase peristalsis, leading to a false interpretation of bowel sounds, and can also reduce compliance of the chid should pain be caused by percussion and palpation.

Using a stethoscope, take the diaphragm end piece and hold it lightly against the skin. A methodical assessment begins in the right lower quadrant slightly below and to the right of the umbilicus (as bowel sounds are normally present here), moving in a clockwise direction throughout the four quadrants.

- Bowel sounds – note the character and frequency of bowel sounds. Normal sounds are high-pitched and gurgling caused by air mixing with fluid during peristalsis. Bowels sounds are generally irregular, occurring between 5 and 35 times per minute. Abnormal bowel sounds include hyperactive sounds which are loud, high-pitched, rushing sounds potentially occurring with early bowel obstruction, gastroenteritis, diarrhoea, Crohn's disease, ulcerative colitis and laxative use. Hypoactive or absent bowel sounds will be evident in complete bowel obstruction or for a period of time following abdominal surgery.
- Vascular sounds – not normally heard but auscultation with the bell end of the stethoscope over the aorta, renal arteries, iliac and femoral arteries should be conducted.

Palpation

Palpation of the abdomen is conducted in two phases. First light palpation is applied, followed by deeper palpation depending on patient tolerance. The aim of palpation is to determine the size, shape, position and tenderness of major abdominal organs and to detect masses and accumulation of fluid (Wolters Kluwer Health 2008).

- Light palpation – hold the four fingers of your dominant hand together and depress the skin about 1–1.5 cm. Make a gentle rotating movement, lift the fingers and move clockwise. The abdomen should be soft and non-tender. Differentiate between resistance from the patient due to them being cold, ticklish or afraid or due to involuntary guarding or rigidity from muscle spasms or peritoneal inflammation. A common finding in children with acute appendicitis is umbilical abdominal pain which then localizes to the right lower quadrant. In children under two years of age the pain of appendicitis is poorly localized and perforation is common (Sondheimer 2004). Peritonitis in children is another diagnosis for consideration when children have acute abdominal pain. Other symptoms include fever, nausea and vomiting with involuntary guarding on palpation.

- Deep palpation – the technique is the same but the abdomen is depressed 5–8 cm. Note the location, size and consistency of any palpable organs. The presence of abnormal enlargement, tenderness or masses should be documented. To palpate the liver ask the child to sit up in bed. Stand on their right side and place your left hand under their back, parallel to the 11th and 12th ribs. Place your right hand in the right upper quadrant and point your fingers down in the direction of the child's head. Ask the child to breathe in and press in and up on the abdomen. You may feel the edge of the liver at your fingertips, which should be smooth and firm. It is common not to locate the liver on palpation. If the liver is palpated 1–2 cm below the right costal margin that it is considered enlarged (Jarvis 2004). The spleen is not normally palpable unless it is enlarged approximately three times its normal size. To palpate the spleen, stand on the patient's right side. Place your left hand over the abdomen to support the posterior left lower rib cage. Place your right hand on the left upper quadrant with fingers facing towards the left axilla. Push your hand deeply down and under the left costal margin. You should not feel anything firm.
- Rectal examination – this may need to be performed to assist with diagnosis but should be done by a qualified member of the surgical team. Rectal examination in a child with acute appendicitis may reveal localized mass or tenderness.

It is important to avoid abdominal palpation of a child presenting with a rigid abdomen. The child may be suffering from peritoneal inflammation and palpation could rupture an inflamed organ. Referral to the appropriate surgical team is essential to ensure timely interventions. As with all systems assessment, documentation of findings is paramount. It may not be possible to diagnose the condition immediately, and repeated abdominal assessment may need to be performed.

Percussion

Percussion is used to determine the size and location of abdominal organs as well as to locate fluid or air present in the abdomen, stomach or bowel.

- General tympany – (a clear hollow sound) is usually present throughout the abdomen as air is present in the stomach and bowel. To determine tympany use the middle finger of your dominant hand to strike a finger resting on the patient's abdomen. Begin in the right lower quadrant and move clockwise through the four quadrants. Dullness occurs over fluid or a mass. Dullness will also be present when percussing organs such as the liver and kidneys. Hyperresonance is present with gaseous distension.

- Liver – percussion can aid in determining liver size. Start in the right midclavicular line in an area of lung resonance and percuss downward towards the liver until the sound changes to a dull quality (usually the 5th intercostal space). Mark the spot. Then commence percussion again in the right midclavicular line at a level below the umbilicus and percuss upwards. Stop when sounds change from tympany to dull and mark the spot. Measure the distance between the two marks.

- Spleen – located at about the level of the 10th rib in the left midaxillary line. Percussion of the spleen is not normally possible due to tympany from the colon although a small area of dullness may be noted. Dullness forward of the midaxillary line indicates enlargement of the spleen. Conditions causing this include trauma, illness that destroys red blood cells such as sickle cell disease, infection and certain liver conditions leading to hepatosplenomegaly.

Nutrition

Children with gastrointestinal malfunction require assessment and monitoring of their nutritional status. As previously described, the gastrointestinal tract and accessory organs are responsible for digestion, absorption, secretion and elimination, including absorption of essential nutrients and vitamins from our diet to maintain a healthy state. When these processes are absent or impaired, practitioners will need to utilize methods to support these bodily functions with the primary aim being to maintain adequate nutritional status. To ensure that this is achieved a nutritional assessment will need to be conducted utilizing the expertise of a paediatric dietician (Bowling 2004).

All children admitted to the high dependency unit should be weighed when feasible and this should be plotted on a growth chart. Growth charts are available for boys and girls up to the age of 18 years and aid visualization of the overall growth progress. Height should also be measured and plotted. In children under the age of two years the measurement of head circumference is often easier and more accurate than height. Weight faltering can be taken generally as a two major centile difference in the height/head circumference plot (Wright et al. 2002). Table 7.3 provides details of the requirements for individual children that are taken into consideration when planning nutritional intake.

Children who are seriously ill, who have liver disease, have suffered burns, have been involved in traumatic accident, suffer inflammatory bowel disease or are experiencing diarrhoea generally have higher nutritional requirements than those detailed in Table 7.3. It is essential

Table 7.3 Nutritional requirements. Source: HMSO (1991). Reproduced with permission *Dietary Reference Values for Food Energy & Nutrients for the United Kingdom. Report of the Panel on Dietary Reference Values of the Committee on Medical Aspects of Food Policy.* Crown copyright DH. RHSS 41.

Age	Fluid (ml/kg)	Energy (kcal/d) (EAR)		Protein (g/d)		Sodium (mmol/d)	Potassium (mmol/d)
		Male	*Female*	*Male*	*Female*		
0–3 m	150	545	515	12.5		9	20
4–6 m	130	690	645	12.7		12	22
7–9 m	120	825	765	13.7		14	18
10–12 m	110	920	865	14.9		15	18
1–3 y	95	1230	1165	14.5		22	20
4–6 y	85	1715	1545	19.7		30	28
7–10 y	75	1970	1740	28.3		50	50
11–14 y	55	2220	1845	42.1		70	80
15–18 y	50	2755	2110	55.2	45.4	70	90

EAR, estimated average requirements

that their nutritional requirements are planned in conjunction with the dietetic team to ensure nutritional intake is adequate. Nursing staff should maintain accurate fluid balance charts to assist the dietician's assessment.

The preferred method of feeding for children who have a functional gastrointestinal tract is the oral or enteral route. Nutritional support via the oral route may include food fortification, sip feeds or energy supplements. Using extra snacks in addition to the hospital menu can encourage a child to increase their daily intake. When the oral route is not an option, feeding is delivered via the enteral route.

The most common method for administering enteral feeding is via a nasogastric (NG) tube. A nasogastric tube is considered a short-term feeding device when gag and coughing reflexes are intact and gastric emptying is adequate (Holmes 2004). Nasogastric tubes can be polyvinyl tubes that remain in situ for up to 1 week and are removed and changed after a week. For children whom it is predicted feeding enterally shall be necessary for periods >1 week, polyurethane or silicone tubes may be utilized as these can be left in place for 30 days. The size of tube chosen will vary dependent on the child's age as well as the consistency of the feed to be administered. A rough guide to tube sizes is infants 6 Fr, toddlers 8 Fr, school-age children 10 Fr and teenagers 12 Fr–14 Fr. The verification of tube position before feeding is essential as feeding into locations other than the stomach may lead to problems with malabsorbtion, diarrhoea, peritonitis and, more seriously, pulmonary aspiration (Sanko 2004). It is estimated that placement of the nasogastric tube into the respiratory tract occurs in 5% of nasogastric tube insertions (Ellett 2004). Patients within the HDU are at a particular high risk of this occurring as they may not display the expected symptoms of respiratory placement due to possible decreased level of consciousness, reduced couch and gag, and recent extubation (Metheny *et al.* 1998). X-ray is considered the gold standard for determining position (Metheney *et al.* 1998; Ellett 2004); however, reducing the exposure of patients to inappropiate amounts of radiation needs to be considered.

The National Patient Safety Agency (2005) issued advice to the health service on reducing harm caused by misplacement of nasogastric tubes. They recommend:

- pH aspirate (stomach contents) should be measured using pH indicator strips in the range of 0–6 with half-point gradients;
- Radiography (x-rays) is recommended but should not be used routinely. Full radio-opaque tubes with markings to enable measurement, identification and documentation of the external lengths should be used.

The following are not recommended:

- The whoosh test which involves the use of a syringe to push a small volume of air down the nasogastric tube whilst sounds produced are monitored by a stethoscope;
- Blue litmus paper;
- Monitoring for bubbling at the end of the tube.

A pH of 0–5.5 confirms gastric placement. A pH 6 or more may indicate bronchial placement and recommendations are that the tube is left in situ for 1 hour and then retested. If aspirate is not obtained or pH is >5.5 the tube should be re-passed or x-ray taken to confirm position. Hospitals usually have local policies in relation to the care of children with nasogastric tubes and these should be followed. A point to note is that some medications (such as omeprazole) may raise gastric and intestinal pH (May 2007), hence a nasogastric tube could be in the correct position but gastric contents would have an alkaline pH. In these circumstances it may be necessary to confirm the tube position on x-ray when it is first passed.

When enteral feeding extends over a longer period (generally >6 weeks) alternative methods of meeting nutritional requirements may need to be considered. In paediatrics it is common for children to have a gastrostomy sited. Gastrostomies are plastic tubes placed directly into the stomach through the abdomen. Gastrostomy tubes may be placed by open surgical techniques, laparoscopy or percutaneously using endoscopy. Percutaneous endoscopic gastrostomy (PEG) has become the technique of choice (Laasch 2003) and it is considered a relatively 'safe' procedure causing minimal pain. Feed is delivered via the gastrostomy tube and may also be used for administration of medication. The device is easily hidden underneath children's clothing and is usually well tolerated. Enteral feeding (even in small amounts) stimulates bile secretion and splanchnic blood flow, maintains intestinal and pancreatic mass, protects against cholestasis and maintains gut barrier function (Bowling 2004; Cerra 1997) and therefore should always be promoted. In some instances, though, enteral feeding may not be achievable.

When children experience impairment of gastrointestinal function it may not be possible to maintain adequate nutrition via the oral or enteral route as adequate absorption of nutrients from the diet is not achievable and malnutrition usually prevails. In clinical practice, alternative methods of feeding such as parenteral nutrition may be recommended. Parenteral feeding requires insertion of a PIC line or central venous line (a Hickman line or Port-a-Cath may be necessary) to aid delivery of nutrients directly into the blood. Common indications for parenteral nutrition in children include short bowel syndrome, necrotizing enterocolitis, congenital abnormalities such as gastroschisis, and gastrointestinal surgery. Children with chronic liver disease may also require parenteral nutrition if establishment of oral/enteral feeding is not achieved or is determined inadequate to maintain growth.

Any child receiving nutritional support needs to be closely monitored by expert members of the multidisciplinary team. Accurate fluid charts need to be maintained by nursing staff. Regular measurement of weight should be taken and documented. Nutritional status should be discussed on ward rounds and close interaction with the dietetic team is essential. Children will also require regular blood samples for biochemistry (particularly if receiving parenteral nutrition) to ensure electrolyte stability. If oral feeding is not possible, liaison with the speech therapy team should be considered to provide oral stimulation to the child. Communication with the child and family is essential to understand feeding patterns and planning of nutritional interventions. Cooperation with feeding regimes is essential if a child is to benefit from nutritional support.

Supporting breastfeeding in a high dependency unit

Breastfeeding is recognized as the best method of feeding infants and the World Health Organization (WHO) recommends exclusive breastfeeding for the first six months of life (WHO 2003). Exclusive breastfeeding means no water, formula or weaning foods. Breastfeeding is the physiological way to feed infants (Lawson 2007) and so all efforts should be made to support breastfeeding if an infant who is breastfed is admitted to the high dependency unit.

Benefits of breastfeeding for sick infants include:

- Protection from allergies, bacterial infections, otitis media and gastrointestinal infections;
- Breast milk is more easily tolerated by sick infants;
- Breastfeeding can have analgesic properties during heel pricks and venepuncture.

It is important that staff in the high dependency unit have the skills and knowledge required to support breastfeeding mothers. In order for breastfeeding to be continued successfully during a period of illness it may mean that the mother will need to express breast milk if the infant is nil by mouth or needs to be tube fed. The unit should have suitable facilities for a mother to express milk. This needs to include the appropriate equipment for expressing breast milk and a designated area for expressing. Some mothers may wish to express at the bedside as they may not want to leave their infant, so this needs to be facilitated by the staff. It is important that mothers are given the correct advice about how often they need to express. It is the frequency of stimulation of the breast that maintains the milk supply rather than the length of time spent on actual expressing (Wallis and Harper 2007). Mothers should be advised to express every three hours in order to maintain their supply during periods when the infant is not feeding (Wallis and Harper 2007). Once expressed the breast milk needs to be stored and handled correctly by the staff. Each Trust should have a policy on the storage and handling of breast milk. Expressed breast milk can be stored for 24 hours but after this time it should be frozen.

In summary, in order for breastfeeding to be successfully supported within the clinical setting the following need to be in place:

- Knowledge of the benefits of breastfeeding;
- Sensitivity and empathy with the breastfeeding mother;
- Knowledge of the physiology of lactation;
- Knowledge of the procedure for the expressing, handling and storage of breast milk (adapted from Wallis and Harper 2007).

Common gastrointestinal conditions

Diabetic ketoacidosis

Diabetic ketoacidosis (DKA) is a potentially life-threatening condition that is caused by absent or insufficient insulin production. Clinical signs of DKA include:

- polyuria
- polydypsia
- vomiting and dehydration

- lethargy and decreased level of consciousness
- hyperventilation
- electrolyte abnormalities
- shock.

Children with DKA need to be treated swiftly. They should be assessed using the ABC approach. If their airway is compromised then they should have an airway inserted and a nasogastric tube passed. Children with severe vomiting should always have a nasogastric tube passed to prevent aspiration pneumonia. Once the airway is secure then the child's breathing needs to be assessed. All children with severe DKA should be given 100% oxygen via a facemask, a cannula should be inserted and the child's level of dehydration should be assessed. This forms the circulatory assessment. They should also be attached to a cardiac monitor to check for arrhythmias. Electrolyte imbalance may lead to rhythm disturbance.

Once the initial assessment has been undertaken then the child will need to be stabilized. Treatment of DKA involves the use of fluid replacement to treat the dehydration and insulin therapy. Fluid replacement is calculated using the formula:

requirement = maintenance + deficit

Deficit (in litres) = % dehydration × body weight (kg) this then needs to be converted into ml. A level of no more than 10% dehydration should be used for the calculation.

Maintenance requirements are as follows:

- age 0–2 years: 80 ml/kg/24 h
- age 3–5 years: 70 ml/kg/24 h
- age 6– 9 years: 60 ml/kg/24 h
- age 10–14 years: 50 ml/kg/24 h
- age over 15 years: 30 ml/kg/24 h.

The amount to be given over the next 48 hours is then calculated by

hourly rate = 48 h maintenance + deficit
              – resuscitation fluid already given/48

Source: NICE (2004)

This calculation is crucial as slow metabolic correction is required to minimize the risk of cerebral oedema. Cerebral oedema can be very serious in DKA and carries a mortality of about 25%. Signs of cerebral oedema include change in Glasgow coma score, headache, slowing of the heart rate, rise in blood pressure, decrease in oxygen saturation and abnormal posturing.

Initially the fluid used should be 0.9% saline with 20 mmol potassium added per 500 ml of fluid. After 6 hours and if the blood sugar and sodium levels have stabilized then the fluid can be altered to 0.45% saline with 5% dextrose (NICE 2004).

Insulin also needs to be administered and this is done by continuous intravenous infusion. The dose of insulin is titrated to the blood sugar level.

The child will need to be closely observed during the initial and ongoing management. Observations that need to be undertaken include:

- Continuous cardiac monitoring;
- Blood pressure, heart rate, respiratory rate, temperature and oxygen saturation;
- Glasgow coma score;
- Fluid balance;
- Measurement of urine output and testing for ketones;
- Hourly blood glucose.

Once the child is stabilized then the insulin is changed to subcutaneous and the child can start to eat and drink normally.

Acute abdominal conditions

Appendicitis

Appendicitis is inflammation of the appendix. It is thought to be caused when the opening to the appendix becomes blocked. The blockage can be caused by mucus or stool. Appendicitis is more common in the older child. The child presents with a history of peri-umbilical pain which then changes to localized right lower quadrant pain. The pain is accompanied by vomiting and a fever. Examination of the child will identify the localized response to the pain. Treatment of appendicitis includes intravenous fluid, pain relief and usually surgical intervention to remove the appendix.

Intussusception

Intussusception is the telescoping of one segment of the intestine into another. It is the most common cause of intestinal obstruction in children under the age of six. Most cases occur in children aged 5 months to 1 year of age and it is more common in boys. It presents with abdominal pain, bile-stained vomit and 'redcurrant jelly stool'. Examination of the child will identify fever and a right-sided abdominal mass in 85% of cases. It is most commonly treated with either a barium enema or an air enema. If this is not successful then it is treated surgically.

Malrotation and volvulus

Malrotation and volvulus are most commonly seen in young infants. It is a developmental abnormality of the bowel where the bowel does not coil correctly in the fetus. Volvulus is a complication of malrotation and occurs when the blood supply to the bowel is cut off due to the malrotation. The condition presents with a history of crying and drawing up of the infant's legs demonstrating that the infant is in pain. The pain is intermittent. There may also be little or no bowel movements, and vomiting. Volvulus is treated surgically as there is a risk of necrosis. The infant will also need to be observed for signs of dehydration.

Incarcerated inguinal hernia

An inguinal hernia occurs in the groin and can be a surgical emergency if it becomes incarcerated. The hernia is diagnosed as incarcerated when it can no longer be reduced manually. These primarily present in infants and the symptoms are irritability due to pain, and vomiting. They can also present with poor feeding and abdominal swelling. The hernia is reduced surgically.

Renal system

Anatomy and physiology

The kidney is vital for maintaining control over the volume and content of the blood. Its key functions are:

- Excretion of waste products;
- Regulation of electrolytes;
- Regulation of plasma pH;
- Regulation of blood pressure by the secretion of rennin from the juxtaglomerular apparatus;
- Activation of vitamin D;
- Production of erythropoietin which stimulates red blood cell production in the bone marrow.

The functional unit of the kidney is the nephron. Each nephron consists of a Bowman's capsule, glomerulus and renal tubules. The production of urine has three phases: glomerular filtration, tubular reabsorption and tubular secretion. Glomerular filtration occurs across the glomerular capillary membrane. Water and solutes are forced across the membrane due to the varying pressure differentials within the Bowman's capsule, the renal tubules and the blood. Tubular reabsorption involves the movement of water and solutes from the renal tubules to the peritubular capillaries. This happens due to a mixture of osmosis and active transportation. Water and solutes are removed at different points along the tubules. This balancing of the absorption of water and sodium is controlled by antidiuretic hormone and aldosterone. The amount of water and solutes reabsorbed is related to the child's fluid balance requirements. Tubular secretion is the movement of substances from the blood into the tubules to be excreted in the urine. Substances such as creatinine, urea, potassium and drugs are secreted. This process plays an important role in the maintenance of the blood pH.

These processes are controlled by the juxtaglomerular apparatus. This is a group of specialized cells which sit between the tubule and the blood supply to the kidney. The cells monitor the sodium and water content within the tubule and adjust the size of the arteriole, so controlling the blood flow into the kidney.

Fluid balance in children

The kidneys play an important role in maintaining normal fluid balance in children but there are other systems that are also involved. Water in body tissues is contained within compartments. Intracellular fluid is water contained within cells and extracellular fluid is water outside of the cells. Extracellular fluid consists of intravascular fluid, interstitial fluid and transcellular fluid (Willock and Jewkes 2000). Infants have a larger proportion of extracellular fluid than older children and this increases their risk of dehydration as extracellular fluid is more easily lost.

Movement of fluids to and from the vascular space into the tissues is dependent upon the following factors:

- osmotic pressure
- oncotic pressure
- hydrostatic pressure
- capillary permeability.

Osmotic pressure relates to the number of particles dissolved in a fluid. A fluid with a low osmotic pressure has a lower concentration of particles dissolved in it. Sodium is the main particle involved in maintaining the osmotic balance in the body. Water moves from an area of low osmotic pressure to an area of high osmotic pressure. What this means in relation to body fluids is that if there is a sudden drop in the level of sodium within the blood (intravascular fluid) due to loss of sodium then water will move from the intravascular space into the tissues (interstitial space). This can lead to problems if this is happening in the cerebral tissues.

Oncotic pressure is the ability of plasma proteins to hold water. Water held by plasma proteins is kept in the intravascular space so helping to maintain intravascular volume.

Hydrostatic pressure is the pressure exerted by water in the blood vessels or tissues. The force of the cardiac contraction causes hydrostatic pressure in the capillaries. This is usually balanced by the hydrostatic pressure in the tissues but in the case of heart failure the hydrostatic pressure in the capillaries is lowered.

Capillary permeability is the ability of the capillaries to allow particles to move across their walls. Usually the openings in the capillary walls are too small to allow the passage of proteins but in some disease processes this becomes impaired. In sepsis capillary permeability increases and proteins are lost through the capillary walls. This leads to the characteristic huge drops in intravascular volume that are seen in sepsis.

All of these factors play a part in ensuring that the balance between intravascular, interstitial and transcellular fluid is maintained. Normal maintenance fluid requirements vary depending upon the age of the child. Neonates have greater fluid requirements than older children. In general the fluid requirements are calculated according to body weight:

- 100 ml/kg day for the first 10 kg of body weight
- 50 ml/kg/day for the second 10 kg of body weight
- 20 ml/kg/day for each additional kg of body weight (Snyder *et al.* 2008).

For example, daily fluid requirements for a child weighing 15 kg would be:

100×10 for first 10 kg

50×10 for second 10 kg

Total fluid requirement: 1500 ml/day or 62 ml/hour.

When assessing hydration in the sick child there are several factors that need to be taken into account. These include:

- the capillary refill time
- the toe–core temperature gap
- the tissue turgor
- the presence of oedema
- the peripheral pulses
- the heart rate
- the mucous membranes
- the urine output
- the body weight.

Other factors such as the child's general appearance and behaviour will also need to be taken into consideration.

Common renal conditions

Dehydration

Children with severe dehydration may need to be treated in a high dependency setting. Dehydration in children is usually isonatraemic, where the serum sodium levels are normal, but in a small number of cases it can be hyponatraemic or hypernatraemic. Dehydration can be caused by a number of different factors including gastroenteritis, DKA, and oral or throat conditions that limit intake due to pain and fever. It is important to assess the level of dehydration accurately so that treatment can be instigated correctly. The most reliable indicators of level of dehydration have been identified as abnormal capillary refill time, abnormal skin turgor and abnormal respiratory pattern (Steiner *et al.* 2004). Clinical assessment of dehydration can be categorized in the following way:

Mild to moderate dehydration:

- Restlessness or irritability
- Sunken eyes
- Thirsty and drinks eagerly
- Mild dehydration: 5–6% loss of body weight.

Severe dehydration:

- Over 10% loss of body weight
- Sunken eyes
- Lethargic or sleepy
- Drinking poorly or not at all.

Skin turgor should be assessed by pinching the skin of the abdomen or the thigh. In normally hydrated children the skin fold retracts immediately, in mild to moderate dehydration it is slow but the skin fold is only visible for 2 seconds; in severe dehydration the skin fold is visible for longer than 2 seconds (Otieno *et al.* 2004).

Once the level of dehydration has been assessed then fluid replacement therapy should be started. A bolus dose of crystalloid fluid should be given to all children with moderate or severe dehydration. This should be 10–20 ml/kg. This dose can be repeated if necessary, then maintenance fluids as previously discussed should be commenced.

Acute renal failure

Children with acute renal failure may be admitted to a high dependency unit prior to their transfer either to a PICU or a renal centre.

Acute renal failure may also occur as a consequence of another illness so it is important to be aware of the signs and symptoms. Acute renal failure results from a sudden loss of renal function accompanied by retention of waste products normally excreted by the kidneys. If treated quickly it is reversible. It can be classified into three groups: prerenal, intrinsic and postrenal. Prerenal failure is the commonest form and the least severe. It is caused by a decrease in the blood supply to the kidneys. This is often the result of shock, cardiac failure, renal artery obstruction or asphyxia. Reduction in blood flow to the kidney results in a reduction in the glomerular filtration rate. Renal function will return with the correction of the problem so treatment is often short-term. Intrinsic renal failure is caused by a problem within the kidney itself. This can be as a result of prerenal failure that is prolonged, leading to poor blood supply for a lengthy period of time. This poor perfusion to the kidney causes damage to the tubules within the kidney. Intrinsic renal failure can also be caused by toxins affecting the kidney such as drug toxicity, coagulation disorders or infection. Necrotic damage is caused to the tubule and renal replacement therapy is required while this damage heals. Permanent damage can be caused requiring transplantation. The final type of acute renal failure is postrenal failure. This is when there is obstruction to the flow of urine. Causes include external masses, blood clots, calculi, inflammation and problems with the urethral valves. Treatment of postrenal failure usually involves surgery, and once the obstruction is removed renal function returns to normal.

Signs and symptoms of acute renal failure include:

- Poor urine output less than 1 ml/kg/h
- Rising serum potassium and phosphate levels
- Rising creatinine levels
- Falling serum sodium, bicarbonate calcium and pH
- Pulmonary oedema
- Peripheral oedema
- High central venous pressure.

Usually a fluid challenge will be given to see if urine output will return; if this is unsuccessful then a diuretic can be administered. If this is also unsuccessful then renal failure can be diagnosed and the child will be placed on fluid restriction. Transfer to an appropriate centre where renal replacement therapy can be instigated is then required.

Below are some case studies examining children presenting with gastrointestinal disorders with diagnosis and treatment options discussed.

Case study 1: 11-year-old with appendicitis

Jimmy, an 11-year-old boy, presents with fever, lethargy, vomiting and abdominal pain.

History: taken from Jimmy and family. Jimmy is normally fit and well. Vomiting began 24 hours ago. Not wanting to eat or drink for 24 hours. Complaining of tummy pain. Fever persistent for 12 hours. Given paracetemol to treat fever and pain.

If Jimmy will cooperate, ask him to sit on the bed to aid examination.

Management

Inspection: Facial grimace as Jimmy gets up onto the bed. Holding right side of abdomen. Feeling tired. Lift clothes to revel abdomen. No bumps, rashes, scars or masses are visible. Skin is pink and smooth. Umbilicus located in middle and inverted. No peristalsis waves are seen.

Auscultation: High-pitched bowel sounds audible in RLQ (note history of diarrhoea). No vascular sounds audible.

Percussion: Tympany throughout the abdomen. Jimmy guards abdomen and asks you to stop when percussing RLQ. When able to carry out further examination with Jimmy's cooperation continue – liver and spleen not felt. Liver borders marked (normal size).

Palpation: Start with light palpation but Jimmy not able to tolerate so examination abandoned.

Routine observations Jimmy is pyrexial 38.2 °C with tachycardia of 120 bpm and a tachypnoea of 24 respirations per minute with an O_2 saturation of 95% in room air.

Following examination, clinical picture suggests an acute abdominal problem with differential diagnosis of Crohn's disease, peritonitis, pneumonia, urinary tract infection and appendicitis, to list a few. Further investigations are required and referral to surgical team made.

Two further tests to include while examining patient to aid diagnosis:

1. *Psoas sign:* the right iliopsoas muscle lies under the appendix when the patient is supine. Inflamed appendix in the retro-

peritoneal location will elicit a positive psoas sign. Ask Jimmy to lie on his left side. Extend his right leg behind him. If pain results this is confirmed as a positive psoas sign and may indicate appendicitis.

2. *Obturator sign:* if appendix is enlarged it may come into contact with the obturator internus muscle. To examine this, lie Jimmy on his back and flex his right hip at a 90° angle. Hold his ankle with your right hand and with your left hand rotate the hip by pulling the knee to and away from Jimmy's body. If pain is elicited, this is a positive obturator sign suggestive of inflamed appendix in pelvis region.

Jimmy demonstrates a positive psoas sign.

Initial intervention

- Administer oxygen by face mask and note effect on oxygen saturations.
- Regular observation of temperature, pulse, blood pressure, respiratory rate and oxygen saturations should be recorded. Use an early warning system if available and report and act on any change in condition.
- Blood tests including FBC, U&E, blood culture and blood glucose should be sent to the laboratory and a cannula should be inserted whilst sampling blood. Analysis shows the white cell count is elevated. Jimmy is pyrexial 38.2 °C with tachycardia at 120 bpm. Electrolytes show low potassium at 3.1 mmol. Intravenous maintenance fluids should be commenced with supplemental electrolytes. Jimmy should remain nil by mouth until reviewed by surgical team.
- Urine sample should be taken and analysed. Urine sample is positive for ketones (no other abnormalities) which rules out UTI.
- Frequent assessment of abdomen should be conducted but be aware of Jimmy's pain. Administer analgesia as required (may need to be given via the IV route).

Management

Surgical team review – conduct abdominal assessment and in conjunction with other findings work on diagnosis of appendicitis. Abdominal ultrasound and computed tomography scans ordered and carried out. Jimmy prepared for exploratory laparotomy and possible removal of appendix.

> ## Case study 2: 3-year-old with diabetic ketoacidosis
>
> A 3-year-old boy presents to the emergency department with abdominal pain, lethargy and vomiting.
> *History:* Taken from family – Generally fit and well. Lost weight over the last few weeks. Bed wetting. Constantly thirsty. Lethargic for 24 hours. Complaining of abdominal pain for 7 hours. No previous visits to hospital. No medications given. Maternal grandfather has diabetes and cardiac problems.

Management

Inspection: Child on parent's knee. Sitting quietly. Drinking cup of water. Talking to family. Breathing quick and deep (respiratory rate 55 bpm). Cracked lips. T-shirt lifted to aid assessment. No bumps, rashes, scars or masses are visible. Skin is pink and smooth. Umbilicus located in middle and inverted. No peristalsis waves are seen.

Auscultation: High-pitched, gurgling bowel sounds audible in RLQ and LLQ. No vascular sounds heard.

Percussion: Normal tympany throughout. No abdominal tenderness with percussion. Liver borders marked (normal size).

Light palpation: Soft, non-tender throughout all quadrants. No abnormalities felt.

Deep palpation: Soft, non-tender throughout all quadrants. Liver and spleen not palpable.

Routine observations: HR 140 bpm, RR 55 bpm, BP 90/50 mmHg, SpO$_2$ 100% in room air, temperature 36.5 °C. Capillary refill 4 seconds centrally and peripherally.

Initial intervention

Additional monitoring (O$_2$ saturations and ECG monitoring), cannula inserted and blood samples taken for FBC, U&E, culture, blood glucose and blood gas.

Immediate results: blood glucose 19 mmol/l (abnormally high). Blood gas analysis pH 7.0, P CO$_2$ 3 kPa, P O$_2$ 11.3 kPa, HCO$_3$ 10, base excess −12 (metabolic acidosis with respiratory compensation).

Bolus of 0.9% saline (10 ml/kg) given over 30 minutes.

Urine sample obtained: tests positive for glucose and ketones.

Working diagnosis of diabetes mellitus presenting in diabetic keto-acidosis. Note the body's natural compensatory mechanism of an elevated respiratory rate to excrete more CO_2 in response to a decreased bicarbonate as the bicarbonate has been used as a buffer for the acidic ketone bodies produced in diabetic ketoacidosis.

Management

As per NICE recommendations (2004) a second cannula inserted. Commence IV fluids (initially 0.9% saline with 20 mmol KCl per 500 ml). Consider calculating fluid deficit and replacing this over 48 hours, (replacing over this time period reduces the likelihood of cerebral oedema occurring from rapid fluid administration). Commence insulin infusion at 0.1 iu/kg/h. Admit patient to paediatric ward.

Record hourly blood glucose (blood glucose levels should not fall by more than 5 mmol per hour). Record neurological observations hourly and maintain accurate fluid balance chart. Monitor 4-hourly U&Es along with blood gas analysis. Blood pH should demonstrate improvement after insulin and fluid commences. Once blood glucose <15 mmol/l change IV therapy to 0.45% saline plus 5% dextrose. Consider reducing insulin to 0.05 iu/kg/h. Urine sample should be frequently monitored for ketones and glucose and this should be documented on fluid chart. While clinical protocols facilitate effective management it is clear that extremely deranged blood gas and vital signs such as in this scenario demonstrate the classic example of a high dependency patient. It is paramount to optimize observation and monitoring, utilize an early warning system, and report and act on any change in condition. Left untreated or treated ineffectively, diabetic ketoacidosis will rapidly progress to coma and death.

Refer patient to endocrinology team for guidance on long-term management and when child is clinically well, drinking, and tolerating food, consider changing to subcutaneous insulin. Child and family education commences on living with type 1 diabetes mellitus.

Conclusion

This chapter has discussed some common conditions affecting the gastrointestinal and renal systems. The gastrointestinal system is responsible for ensuring that the body has a constant energy supply to meet the high demands. Compromising of the gastrointestinal tract and accessory organs, its many functions have been detailed above. Disturbances of the functions of the gastrointestinal and renal systems can lead to a chid becoming seriously ill and advanced assessment skills are required from a practitioner if they are to diagnosis and implement effective treatment. Several common problems relating to paediatrics have been discussed and common symptoms related to these highlighted.

Learning activities

- Review case study 1 and discuss how Jimmy would have deteriorated and then further management if observations and interventions had not been instigated in a timely manner.
- Write a care plan for a 15-year-old who has been admitted with suspected diabetic ketoacidosis. Consider acute management and the longer-term psychosocial aspects of being a teenager with a chronic condition.
- Formulate a discussion on the benefits of enteral feeding versus parenteral feeding, considering nutrition, staffing, patient and family, and cost.
- Consider the stigma that a child who suffers from diabetes may encounter and what education could be provided to schools to prevent this.

References and further reading

Bowling T (2004) *Nutritional Support for Adults and Children: a handbook for hospital practice*. Radcliffe Medical Press Ltd, Oxford.

Cerra F (1997) Applied Nutrition in ICU Patients. A Consensus Statement of the American College of Chest Physicians. *Chest* **111**(3): 769–778.

Cooks A (ed.) (2000) *Nutritional Requirements for Children in Health and Disease*. Great Ormond Street Hospital for Children, London.

Ellett MLC (2004) What is known about methods of correctly placing gastric tubes in adults and children? *Gastrointestinal Nursing* **27**(6): 253–259.

Gill D, O'Brien N (2004) *Paediatric Clinical Examination Made Easy*, 4th Edition. Churchill Livingstone, Eindurgh.

Jarvis C (2004) *Pocket Companion for Physical Examination and Health Assessment*, 4th Edition. W.B. Saunders, Philadelphia.

Holmes S (2004) Enteral feeding and percutaneous endoscopic gastrostomy. *Nursing Standard* **18**(20): 41–43.

Kindlen S (2003) *Physiology for Health Care and Nursing*. Churchill Livingstone, Edinburgh.

Laasch H (2003) Gastrostomy Insertion: Comparing the Options: PEG, RIG or PIG? *Clinical Radiology* **58**(5): 398–405.

Lawson M (2007) Contemporary aspects of infant feeding. *Paediatric Nursing* **19**(2): 39–45.

Long C (2002) *Gastrointestinal System*, 2nd Edition. Mosby, St Louis, MO, and London.

May S (2007) Testing nasogastric tube positioning in the critically ill: exploring the evidence. *British Journal of Nursing* **16**(7): 414–418.

Metheny NA, Wehrle MA, Wiersema L, Clark J (1998) Testing feeding tube placement: auscultation vs pH method. *American Journal of Nursing* **98**(5): 37–42.

National Institute for Clinical Excellence (2004) *Type 1 Diabetes: Diagnosis and Management of Type 1 Diabetes in Children and Young People*. NICE, London.

National Patient Safety Agency (2005) *Reducing the Harm Caused by Misplaced Nasogastric Feeding Tubes. Interim Advice for Health Care Staff.* February 2005. NPSA, London.

Nursing Standard (2001) Essential Skills. Nutrition and hydration: nasogastric tube insertion. *Nursing Standard* **15**(51).

Otieno H, Were E, Ahmed I (2004) Are bedside features of shock reproducible between different observers? *Archives of Disease in Childhood* **89**(10): 977–979.

Patton K (2006) *Survival Guide for Anatomy and Physiology*. Mosby, St Louis, MO.

Smith G, Watson R (2005) *Gastrointestinal Nursing*. Blackwell Publishing, Oxford.

Sanko J (2004) Aspiration assessment and prevention in critically ill enterally fed patients: evidence-based recommendations for practice. *Gastrointestinal Nursing* **27**(6): 279–285.

Snyder C, Spilde T, Rice H (2008) Fluid Management for the Pediatric Surgical Patient. http://emedicine.medscape.com/article/936511-overview (accessed 21 January 2009).

Sondheimer JM (2004) Gastrointestinal Tract. In Hay WM, Hayward AR, Levin MJ, Sondheimer JM. *Current Pediatric Diagnosis and Treatment*, 17th Edition. McGraw-Hill, New York. Chapter 20.

Steiner MJ, Dewalt DA, Byerley JS (2004) Is this child dehydrated? *Journal of the American Medical Association* **291**(22): 2746–2754.

Wallis M, Harper M (2007) Supporting breastfeeding mothers in hospital. *Paediatric Nursing* **19**(8): 31–35.

Watson R (2005) *Anatomy and Physiology for Nurses*, 12th Edition. Elsevier, Edinburgh.

Waugh A, Grant A (2006) *Ross and Wilson. Anatomy and Physiology in Health and Illness*. Elsevier, Edinburgh.

Weber J, Kelley J (2006) *Health Assessment in Nursing*, 3rd Edition. Philadelphia: Lippincott Williams & Wilkins.

Whiteman K, McCormick C (2005) When your patient is in liver failure. *Nursing* **35**(4): 58–63.

Willick J, Jewkes F (2000) Making sense of fluid balance in children. *Paediatric Nursing* **12**(7): 37–42.

Wolters Kluwer Health (2008) *Assessment Made Incredibly Easy*, 4th Edition. Lippincott Williams & Wilkins, New York.

World Health Organization (2003) *Global Strategy for Infant Feeding*. WHO, Geneva.

Wright CM, Booth IW, Buckler JMH (2002) Growth Reference Charts for use in the United Kingdom. *Archives of Disease in Childhood* **86**: 11–14.

The immunocompromised child

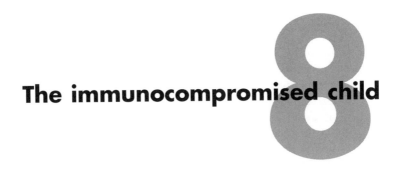

Joan Walters

Learning outcomes

- To develop an understanding of the normal physiology of the immune system by the end of the chapter
- To develop an understanding of the clinical features of infection
- To develop an understanding of the prevention of the spread of infection
- To develop an understanding of the management of infection

Introduction

Infectious diseases are still a major cause of mortality and morbidity in the modern developed world. Daily we are learning more about the complexity of the immune system. Children, because of their young age and the immaturity of their immune systems, are particularly susceptible to infections that are prevented in older patients through vaccination or via a more robust, innate immune response (Posfay-Barbe *et al.* 2008). Although community-acquired infection represents the bulk of all infection seen in both primary and secondary care, the transmission of infection in or during health care (healthcare-acquired infection, HAI) has now become extremely important in the ongoing care of patients (Todd *et al.* 2006).

Close physical contact between children in communal rooms or play areas, between children and visitors such as parents and siblings, and uncontrolled fluids and bodily secretions also provide ample opportunities for the spread of infection. Specific aspects of children's hospitals, such as shared rooms in general paediatric intensive care units (PICUs) or high dependency units (HDU) instead of separate medical and surgical ICUs/HDUs as for adults, toy-sharing, pet-visiting, and partial ambulatory care, also contribute to the risk of nosocomial infection (Posfay-Barbe *et al.* 2008). Other risk factors for HAI include close physical contact with healthcare workers and staying in environments where antibiotic-resistant organisms are endemic. Thus, the close proximity of compromised patients in the hospital setting, coupled with the concentrated use of antibiotics and the ease of transmission by healthcare workers, has led to the selection of multidrug-resistant organisms such as MRSA, vancomycin-resistant enterococci (VRE) and extended spectrum β-lactamase resistant (ESBL) bacteria. In addition, the easy spread of organisms such as these, plus infections such as *Clostridium difficile* and norovirus, may lead to outbreaks of infection that can only be contained by ward or hospital closure (Todd *et al.* 2006).

A nosocomial infection is an infection acquired in a hospital – specifically, an infection that was not present or incubating prior to the patient being admitted to the hospital, but occurred within 72 hours after admittance to the hospital (Department of Health 2004). HAIs affect approximately 10% of all hospital admissions and create a significant burden both clinically and economically (Department of Health 2004). In both adults and children, certain patients are particularly at risk of HAIs; among these are those patients with a low white cell count and those in intensive and high dependency care settings with indwelling devices.

This chapter will explore normal physiology of the immune system, how infections enter the body, factors that increased susceptibility, and how to prevent infections or how to manage an infection once it has been acquired.

Clinical examination

The possible indicators of an acute infection are:

- Fever which is associated with anorexia, protein catabolism, negative nitrogen balance, acute phase protein response, hypoalbuminaemia, low serum iron, sequestration of iron, anaemia and neutrophilia (Griffin *et al.* 1999). This is due to a resetting of the thermostat in the anterior hypothalamus to a higher setting – a purposeful reaction, potentiating the immune and inflammatory response to infection (Southgate *et al.* 1997);

- Convulsion, especially in young children;
- Fatigue;
- Haemorrhage, haemolytic anaemia and intravascular coagulation;
- Headache;
- Lymph node enlargement;
- Malaise;
- Nausea and vomiting;
- Organ failure, e.g. heart, brain, lung, liver and necrosis of the skin;
- Rash – a common feature of many systemic infectious diseases, e.g. measles, meningococcal infection, rubella;
- Shock – sustained fall in circulating blood volume associated with lowered system reaction;
- Tachycardia;
- Tachypnoea (Whittaker 2004; Griffin *et al.* 1999).

If a localized infection is suspected, possible indicators may be:

- Redness and swelling due to vasodilation;
- Swelling or oedema due to increased vascular permeability;
- Pain or tenderness caused by chemical mediators and pressure from increased tissue fluids;
- Possible restricted movement of a body part;
- Possible drainage from open lesions or wounds (Whittaker 2004).

Normal physiology

The immune system operates throughout the body. Its main function is the identification and destruction of antigens. It has evolved as a complex network of molecules, cells and organs to defend against pathogenic micro-organisms and non-infectious foreign substances. Beyond its role in host protection, it regulates tissue homeostasis and tissue repair by screening cell surfaces for the expression of specific molecules (Goronzy and Weyand 2009).

Cells of the immune system identify and remove injured, dead, or malignant cells. These substances are capable of interacting with the host's specific immune response causing a specific response (disease). Immune defences are normally categorized into the innate immune response, which provides immediate protection against an invading pathogen, and the adaptive or acquired immune response, which takes more time to develop but confers exquisite specificity and long-lasting protection (Boon *et al.* 2006; Southgate *et al.* 1997). The properties of these two types of immune response are listed in Table 8.1.

Table 8.1 Properties of the immune responses. Adapted from Boon *et al.* (2006)

Innate (non-specific) response	Adaptive (specific) response
Skin	
Mucous membranes	
Recognizes generic microbial structures	Antigen-specific responses
Immediately mobilized (minutes)	Slow response (days)
No memory	Memory
Genetically encoded	Not genetically encoded
Essentially identical responses in all individuals	Acquired as an adaptive response to exposure to antigen
Present in invertebrates and vertebrates	Present in invertebrates only

The key components of the immune system to be explored are:

- constitutive barriers (e.g. skin, sweat, mucous membrane)
- phagocytes
- natural killer cells
- soluble mediators, e.g. complement
- T- and B-lymphocytes
- secreted molecules, e.g. antibody
- antigenic specific response.

Constitutive barriers

The tightly packed, highly keratinized cells of the skin constantly undergo renewal and replacement; the tight junctions between cells prevent the majority of pathogens from entering the body. Microbial growth is inhibited by physiological factors such as low pH and low oxygen tension, and sebaceous glands secrete hydrophobic oils that further repel water and micro-organisms. Endogenous commensal bacteria provide an additional constitutive defence against infection. Approximately 100 trillion (10^{14}) bacteria normally reside at epithelial surfaces in symbiosis with the human host. They increase the protective properties of the skin through the secretion on to its surface of bactericidal fatty acids; eradication of the normal flora with broad-spectrum antibiotics commonly results in opportunistic infection by organisms which rapidly colonize an undefended ecological niche (Whittaker 2004).

Sweat also contains lysozyme, an enzyme that destroys the structural integrity of bacterial cell walls; ammonia, which has antibacterial properties; and several antimicrobial peptides such as defensins (Griffin *et al.* 2003; Goronzy and Weyand 2009).

Similarly, the mucous membranes of the respiratory, gastrointestinal and genitourinary tracts provide a constitutive barrier to infection. For example, within the respiratory tract, cilia directly trap pathogens and contribute to removal of mucus, assisted by physical manoeuvres such as sneezing and coughing. Again, within the gastrointestinal tract, hydrochloric acid and salivary amylase chemically destroy bacteria, while normal peristalsis and induced vomiting or diarrhoea promote clearance of invading organisms.

Generally constitutive barriers are highly effective, but if external defences are breached by a wound (including insertion of medical devices, e.g. chest drain, intravenous cannula) or pathogenic organism, the specific soluble proteins and cells of the innate immune system are activated.

Specific immune structures

There are certain sites where the cells of the immune system are organized into specific structures. Immune cells derive from haematopoietic stem cells in the bone marrow circulate in the blood and lymph, forming complex microstructures in specialized lymphoid organs, and infiltrate virtually every tissue. Their anatomic organization in lymphoid organs and their ability to circulate throughout the body and to migrate between blood and lymphoid tissues are crucial components of host defence (Goronzy and Weyand 2009). They are classified as central lymphoid tissue (from the bone marrow and the thymus) and peripheral lymphoid tissue (lymph nodes, spleen, mucosa-associated lymphoid tissue – tonsils, adenoids and appendix).

Lymph nodes (glands) are masses of lymphoid tissue which lie along the course of lymphatic vessels and which filter the lymph. They vary in size from 1 mm to 10 mm and are most numerous in the axillae, groin, neck and posterior wall of the abdominal cavity. Lymphocytes are mainly produced in the lymph nodes.

The thymus gland is found in the thorax in the anterior mediastinum. It gradually enlarges during childhood but after puberty it undergoes a process of involution resulting in a reduction in the functioning mass of the gland.

The following cell types are present:

- lymphoid cells
- epithelial cells
- macrophages
- other supporting cells.

In the thymus gland lymphoid cells undergo a process of maturation and education prior to release into the circulation. This process allows T cells to develop the important attribute known as self tolerance.

Immature lymphoid cells enter the cortex proliferate, mature and pass on to the medulla. From the medulla, mature T lymphocytes enter the circulation.

The thymus continues to function throughout life; however, thymic epithelial cells have different appearances in different locations within the gland.

The spleen is located in the upper left quadrant of the abdomen. It has two main functions and is divided into two distinct components, the red and white pulp.

Acting as part of the immune system, the white pulp consists of aggregates of lymphoid tissue and is responsible for the immunological function of the spleen. Lymphocytes and monocytes are produced here (Griffin et al. 2004).

The white blood cells can be divided into two broad groups, the phagocytes and the immunocytes. Granulocytes, which include three types of cells – neutrophils, esonophils and basophils – together with monocytes, make up the phagocytes. The lymphocytes, their precursor cells and plasma cells make up the immunocytes. They work closely with two soluble protein systems, immunoglobulin and complement, in protecting the body against infection (Hoffbrand et al. 2006).

Neutrophils are the most important phagocytes. They have a very short half-life (6–10 hours). They are able to identify and immobilize an antigen (chemotaxis), ingest the antigen (phagocytosis) and kill and digest an antigen. If their numbers are low a person is said to be neutropenic. Neutropenia increases risk of infection and this risk increases as depth and length of neutropenia increases. Diapedesis (the ability of the cells to move) in an amoeboid fashion and changing shape to move between epithelial cells and into tissue is important, and not well developed in infants (Purssell 2004; Randall 2004; Whittaker 2004).

T-cells (lymphocytes) are the key immunocytes and have two major roles in immune defence. First, regulatory T-cells are essential for orchestrating the response of an elaborate system of different types of immune cells. Helper T-cells, for example, also known as CD4 positive T-cells (CD4+ T-cells), alert B-cells (lymphocytes) to start making antibodies; they also can activate other T-cells and immune system scavenger cells called macrophages, and influence which type of antibody is produced. Certain T-cells, called CD8 positive T-cells (CD8+ T-cells), can become killer cells that attack and destroy infected cells. The killer T-cells are also called cytotoxic T-cells or CTLs (cytotoxic lymphocytes) (Purssell 2004).

Monocytes (macrophages) become important after about 24 hours. They generate C-reactive protein –which is a marker of bacterial disease.

They are part of the complement system, attacking bacteria and acting as an opsonin (molecule that makes an antigen more attractive to phagocytes) (Hoffbrand *et al.* 2006; Purssell 2004).

The complement system is a group of more than 20 tightly regulated, functionally linked proteins that act to promote inflammation and eliminate invading pathogens. Complement proteins are produced by the liver, and are present in the circulation as inactive molecules. When triggered, they activate other proteins in a rapidly amplified biological cascade analogous to the coagulation cascade.

Cytokines are small, secreted, soluble proteins that act as multipurpose chemical messengers. They act locally via cell-specific receptors as part of the innate and adaptive immune response. More than 100 cytokines have been described, with overlapping, complex roles in modifying the immune microenvironment. Subtle differences in cytokine composition, particularly at the initiation of an immune response, may have a major effect on outcome. Some important cytokines include IL-1 involved in fever production and T-cell and macrophage activation and IFN interferon that inhibit virus multiplication within cells (Whittaker 2004).

Pathophysiology

When we think of the problems of the immune system we must consider those who we consider to be at risk. The nosocomial pathogens and most common HAI sites in children differ from those reported among adults. Children have fewer chronic or degenerative organ system disorders than adults but present more often with congenital or acquired immune deficiencies as well as congenital syndromes (Posfay-Barbe *et al.* 2008). Children and the elderly are more susceptible to bacterial pneumonia and intestinal infections. Immunological immunity steadily develops in the first few years of life but diminishes after the age of 45 years when the thymus begins to atrophy and there is a decrease in hormone production which is essential for lymphocyte differentiation (Whittaker 2004). This person is known as the susceptible host. We can then look at why they may lack this is resistance in two ways:

1. They may be *immunocompromised* – having a weakened immune system from whatever cause, e.g. inherited and acquired disorders such as aplastic anaemia, sickle cell disease or diabetes. Trauma, e.g. wounds or burns, open up the skin surface. Certain infections can decrease the individual's resistance to secondary infection, e.g. AIDS;

2. They may be receiving *immunosuppressants* – there is an artificial weakening of an immune system as part of medical treatment, e.g. many of the drugs used to treat childhood cancer or drugs used after organ transplantation can cause immune system and bone marrow suppression. Children may receive drugs to treat autoimmune disease such as rheumatoid arthritis or inflammatory bowel disease (Whittaker 2004; Goronzy and Weyand 2009).

Therefore, there are several key predisposing factors to infection, which will be explored further in the case studies, namely:

- age
- nutritional imbalance
- gender and hormonal factors
- stress
- trauma
- infection and other underlying diseases
- drugs invasive procedures and devices
- local factors
- genetics
- inadequate defences (Whittaker 2004).

It is important to remember that each individual plays host to certain bacteria in specific parts of the body and this is known as normal flora. Sometimes colonization can occur (the presence of bacteria or other organisms) without multiplication and damage to the host tissue (Griffin *et al.* 1999; Whittaker 2004). Therefore, there must be a combination of factors which allow an infection to take hold, including the susceptible host, and also a causative agent, a reservoir, a portal of exit, a mode of infection and a portal of entry. This is known as the cycle of infection (Figure 8.1, Whittaker 2004).

The *causative agents* can be classified as:

1. Bacteria (includes *Rickettsia, Chlamydia, Mycoplasma, Pneumoccocus, Streptococcus, Staphylococcus aureus* and *Escherichia coli*). They are the most significant and most commonly observed in healthcare settings (Whittaker 2004);
2. Viruses (includes rubella);
3. Fungi rarely infect humans unless(includes aspergillums, thrush (Candida) and ringworm);
4. Protozoa (includes malaria, amoebic dysentery and trichomoniasis);
5. Helminths – worm-like animals, parasites (includes roundworm, pinworm (threadworm) and tapeworm).

Causative agents are characterized by the infective dose, pathogenicity, virulence, invasiveness, host specificity, viability, antigenic variation and resistance.

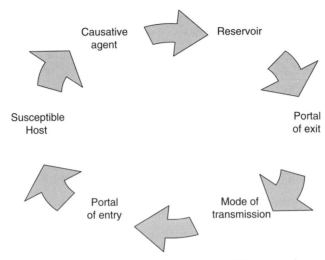

Figure 8.1 The chain of infection. Source: Whittaker N (2004) *Disorders and Interventions*. By kind permission of Palgrave Macmillan.

Table 8.2 Reservoirs of infection. Source: Southgate *et al.* (1997)

Reservoir	
Humans: Patients Healthcare workers Visitors	With an active infection, convalescent but excreting organism, or a symptomless carrier
Animals including insects and rodents	With an active infection, convalescent but excreting organism, or a symptomless carrier, or via an arthropod vector
Environment Patient care equipment Environmental surfaces Food, e.g. egg, shellfish, meat, salad vegetables	Airborne, soils, contaminated food or water

Table 8.2 lists the *reservoirs of infection* to be taken into account. The portals of exit include:

1. Respiratory tract – coughing, sneezing, talking;
2. Genitourinary tract – sexually transmitted diseases and urinary tract infection;
3. Gastrointestinal tract – faeces and vomitus;
4. Skin/mucous membranes – wounds and skin breaks;

5. Transplacental (to foetus from mother);
6. Blood – needlestick injury and blood transfusion.

The *portals of entry* can include all the portals of exit described above. For example:

1. Respiratory tract – suctioning;
2. Genitourinary tract – Foley catheters;
3. Gastrointestinal tract;
4. Skin/mucous membrane – surgical sites, wound sites, trauma sites;
5. Transplacental;
6. Parenteral (percutaneous, e.g. intravenous cannulation, via blood.

The *modes of transmission* are described in Table 8.3.

Through the description of the cycle of infection it can be seen that potential sites for infection include those in which medical equipment such as catheters or drains can be sited:

- respiratory
- bone and joint
- central nervous system
- gastrointestinal system
- skin and soft tissue
- bloodstream
- urinary system (UTI)
- cardiovascular
- eye/ear/throat/mouth infection
- reproductive system.

Table 8.3 Modes of transmission. Source: Southgate *et al.* (1997)

Direct: immediate transmission	Person-to-person Actual physical contact between source and patient
Indirect: patient to contaminated indirect object	Contaminated, e.g. an endoscope Droplets spread (large particles that rapidly settle out on horizontal surfaces – usually within 3 feet of source)
Airborne: organisms contained within droplet nuclei or dust particles	E.g. droplet nuclei of tuberculosis suspended in air for extended periods, may be spread through ventilation systems
Vectorborne: external vector-borne transmission	Mechanical transfer of microbes on external appendages (e.g. the feet of flies)
Harboured by vector	But no biological interaction between vector and agent (e.g. yellow fever virus)

Infection of patients during their care and treatment is common and in some cases life threatening (Department of Health 2004). Therefore, an understanding of all of these factors can enable the nurse to minimize the risk of the transmission of infection.

Investigations

After the physical assessment of the child the most important test is the differential white cell count (WCC) which might be able to confirm presence of an infection or the reason why an infection has taken hold. A raised WCC is known as leucocytosis and is usually indicative of an infection; WCC can be raised in certain allergic reactions or malignancies. A low WCC is known as leucopenia. The platelets are also considered in this test as they may react and become raised in the presence of an infective organism (thrombocytosis). Healthy infants and children <5 years have a higher proportion and concentration of lymphocytes than adults (Provan et al. 2004).

Table 8.4 presents the percentages as being the norm for 90% of the population (mean ±2 standard deviations).

Other common blood tests are the C-reactive protein and the erythrocyte sedimentation rate (ESR), a non-specific test that measures the rate at which red blood cells settle, which is increased in infection and inflammation (Whittaker 2004).

Other investigations are dependent on the suspected site of infection and may include taking a swab from the ears, nose or throat as well as wounds, midstream specimen of urine, faeces or a lumbar puncture to obtain cerebrospinal fluids.

Table 8.4 The differential white count. Source: Griffin et al. (2003) Crash Course in Immunology, 2nd Edition. By kind permission of Elsevier.

Parameters	Normal range	Diagnostic inference
White cell count	$4–11 \times 10^9/l$	↑(leucocytosis)↓ (leucopenia)
Neutrophils	$2–7.7 \times 10^9/l$ (40–80%)	↑(neutrophilia) ↓(neutropenia)
Lymphocytes	$1.3–3.5 \times 10^9/l$ (20–40%)	↑(lympocytosis) ↓(lymphopenia)
Monocytes	$0.2–0.8 \times 10^9/l$ (2–10%)	↑(monocytosis)
Esonophils	$0.04–0.44 \times 10^9/l$ (1–6%)	↑(esonophilia)
Basophils	$0–0.1 \times 0^9/l$ (<1–2%)	↑(basophilia)
Platelets	$150–400 \times 10^9/l$	↑(reactive thrombocytosis): haemorrhage, infection, malignancy, inflammation; or pathological thrombocythaemia); myeloproliferative disorders

Case study 1: 3-year-old with sickle cell disease

Michael Anwa is 3 years old and has sickle cell disease. He was identified by his local screening programme when he was just 3 weeks old. He is in the children's outpatient clinic for a follow-up appointment after a recent admission for pneumonia. The specialist nurse spent some time with his parents to find out if there was any particular reason why Michael had contracted this infection. One of the things that the nurse established was that Michael had not been given his prophylactic treatment of twice daily penicillin. This was because the parents were concerned about the long-term effect of the prophylactic antibiotic but also because Michael did not like the taste of his medication.

Management

On hearing these concerns the nurse felt it was necessary to explain why the medication was important for a child with sickle cell disease. She explained that a child with sickle cell disease (SCD) is immuno-compromised for two reasons: the white blood cells only partially fight infection and the spleen is only partially effective. Infection is the commonest cause of death in children under the age of 2 years with sickle cell disease in developing countries where there is no or limited access to antibiotics (Serjeant and Serjeant 2001).

The usual prophylactic dose of penicillin is:

- 0–5 years – 62.5 mg twice a day;
- 5–12 years- 25 mg twice a day;
- 12 years upwards – 250 mg twice a day.

If a child is allergic to penicillin, erythromycin is used.

The limited ability to fight infection is because the neutrophils' ability to produce opsonins is reduced therefore bacteria and viruses which a healthy individual is able to eradicate can be life threatening. Septicaemia and bacteraemia can occur particularly in the presence of *Pneumonococcus, Haemophilus influenzae, Salmonella* and parvovirus. *Pneumococcus* and *H. influenzae* can lead to life-threatening pneumonia and meningitis, respectively, while *Salmonella* and parvovirus are associated with osteomyelitis and aplastic crisis, respectively. It is known that a child with sickle cell disease is 600 times more likely than the general population to contract a pneumococcal infection. Also the spleen's ability to function is compromised by the sickle-shaped red blood cells damaging the spleen over time, as they go through the spleen to be filtered, like all blood cells (Serjeant and Serjeant 2001).

The nurse goes on to explain that luckily the NHS Newborn Screening programme had picked up Michael's condition so early. Early identification of SCD detection allows for the initiation of prophylactic antibiotics treatment before the age of 3 months. This decreases the frequency of infections and associated morbidity. It is important to remember that the daily dose of penicillin is not a therapeutic dose (a dose sufficient to completely kill off an organism). Therefore, a medical assessment should always be sought for the child who is unwell and has sickle cell disease (Oni *et al.* 2006).

It is recommended that the child with SCD should receive all the vaccinations in the UK Childhood Immunization Programme.

Case study 2: 7-year-old with acute lymphoblastic leukaemia

Alice Mahoney is 7 years old and has acute lymphoblastic leukaemia, a cancer of the blood. She is currently in hospital under barrier protection (protective isolation) because she experienced a febrile neutropenic episode and was unwell. If febrile but well, Alice might have been managed in the community (Phillips *et al.* 2007). She is receiving intravenous antibiotics via a central venous catheter.

Management

Although Alice's infection might have been obtained via several ports of entry, e.g. the respiratory or gastrointestinal tract; it is important to remember a major complication of the use of tunnelled central vascular catheter (TCVC) is infection. The prolonged TCVC access has become necessary for a large number of patients who require parenteral nutrition, chemotherapy, blood products, or antimicrobial therapy. These infections can lead to serious morbidity and death, especially in paediatric oncology patients.

TCVCs should be used in conjunction with the recommendations on 'standard principles'. These recommendations are divided into four intervention categories:

- education of patients, their carers and healthcare personnel
- general asepsis
- catheter site care
- standard principles for catheter management.

Febrile neutropenia can be described as a child having a single temperature greater than a 'peak' (the primary definition) or a prolonged fever of lower intensity (the secondary definition). Most commonly it is 'peak recorded temperature of 38.5°C or two readings of 38°C over the course of 1 hour'. Neutropenia is defined more consistently as an absolute neutrophil count of <1.0×10^9/l (Phillips *et al.* 2007).

In a well person, neutrophils account for 70% of the white cell total. However, with cancer the most common treatment is cytotoxic drug therapy (cell-killing drugs). Unfortunately, these drugs are not able to distinguish between healthy and unhealthy cells and will kill them all. Cancer treatment relies on the fact that the unhealthy cells take longer to recover than healthy cells. This is why the treatment is given in stages, to allow the healthy cells time to recover. However, the healthy cells level may fall so low that sometimes they affect normal body functioning, in this case all of the cells of the bone marrow (myelosuppression).

Management of febrile neutropenia takes account of the common organisms causing infection in this patient group. First-line choice of antibiotic is usually a combination of an aminoglycoside (gentamicin or tobramycin) and a piperacillin-based antibiotic or an aminoglycoside and a cephalosporin (ceftazidime/ceftriaxone or cefuroxime) If significantly unwell a single agent, carbapentane, may be added to an additional aminoglycoside (Phillips *et al.* 2007).

Barrier protection is designed to prevent infection in a compromised and highly susceptible individual. It is used when patients:

- have diseases such as leukaemia, which depress resistance to infections;
- are receiving chemotherapy or radiation therapy;
- are taking immunosuppressive medications, e.g. after transplantation (solid or organ);
- have extensive burns, dermatitis, or other skin impairments that prevent adequate coverage with dressings.

Generally these patients are most at risk from their own resident flora (endogenous infection) but must also be protected from the risk of cross-infection (exogenous infection). These patients may also receive prophylactic antifungals and/or antibiotics to reduce the risk of endogenous infection. The decision to institute protective isolation is made by the clinician caring for the patient or on the advice of the infection control team. The amount of protection required varies with the type of patient. Essentially, such patients should be isolated with a minimum of dust, dirt and wet areas (Alothman 2005).

The basic principles of barrier protection include:

- Single room with doors kept closed. Maximum protective isolation would require the use of a ventilated room or positive pressure isolator and is preferable in severely immunocompromised patients (Phillips *et al.* 2007);
- Hands to be washed on entering and leaving the room;
- Gloves (sterile) to be worn when dealing with intravenous lines, urinary catheters or wounds;
- Aprons to be worn when dealing with wounds or body fluids;
- Members of staff or visitors with known or possible infections must not enter room without discussion with a member of the infection control team;
- Staff nursing patients in protective isolation should not also nurse patients in source isolation, to reduce the risk of spread of infection, from patients with infections to susceptible individuals;
- Toys with cleanable surfaces;
- Patient charts kept outside room;
- Foot-operated pedal bin;
- Ensure food is cooked (avoid fresh fruit and vegetables and non-processed dairy food;
- Avoid fresh flowers and plants.

Further precautions may be necessary following discussion with the infection control team, e.g. the use of sterile water, daily damp dusting or the use of masks (Alothman 2005; Dix 2005).

Case study 3: 12-year-old with peritonitis

Adam Johnson is 12 years old and was brought in to the Emergency Department after having collapsed at home. He had been complaining of intermittent right lower quadrant pain for a few days and had stayed away from school the day prior to his admission. He had also been off his food, complaining of nausea, and had been vomiting for one day. He has no other history of significant ill health.

Management

On presentation, history and physical examination suggested peritonitis secondary to a ruptured inflamed appendix (appendicitis). This allows for the entry of bacteria or enzymes into the peritoneum (the abdominal cavity). This lead to peritonitis, a serious inflammation of the abdominal cavity's lining (the peritoneum) that can be fatal unless it is treated quickly. Therefore, appendicitis is considered to be a medical emergency that requires prompt surgery to remove the appendix (appendectomy).

Adam did not demonstrate many of the classic signs as his appendix had already ruptured. Many children do not manifest some of the common signs and are therefore more likely to present when their appendix has ruptured or has formed an abscess (Humes and Simpson 2006). However, Adam did demonstrate some of the later signs, a fever with chills, beginning after other symptoms, and abdominal swelling, as well as increased breathing and heart rates, shallow breaths, low blood pressure and limited urine production.

These latter signs along with warm peripheries and a raised white cell count are traditionally indicative of sepsis, with the implication that the clinical picture is caused by invading micro-organisms and their breakdown products. However, other conditions such as pancreatitis, trauma, malignancy, tissue necrosis, aspiration syndromes, liver failure, blood transfusion and drug reactions can all produce the same clinical picture in the absence of infection (Treacher and Grant 2006).

Adam is immunocompromised through a period of anorexia, the entry of bacteria into his abdominal cavity, and poorly perfused tissue. There is also the physical stress of surgery and the resultant need for several ports of entry (surgical wound and intravenous cannula). Septic shock is the clinical manifestation of overwhelming inflammation. Failure of normal inhibitory mechanisms results in excessive production of proinflammatory cytokines by macrophages.

Without surgery or antibiotics, mortality is >50%. With early surgery, the mortality rate is <1%, and convalescence is normally rapid and complete. With complications (rupture and development of an abscess or peritonitis), the prognosis is worse: repeat operations and a long convalescence may follow (Humes and Simpson 2006).

Not eating for several days can rapidly lead to nutritional imbalance. Lymphoid tissue is vulnerable to excesses and deficiencies of many nutrients. Starvation preoperatively leads to a state of catabolism and can have detrimental effects on the patient. The onset of starvation results in a decrease in the absorption of glucose, amino acids and fatty acids from the intestine. During surgery the body increases its use of energy but its nutritional intake decreases (Callaghan 2002). Without the required nutrients and energy for the production of antibodies, lymphocytes and the chemical mediators, the immune response is impaired.

Treatment

Appendectomy should be preceded by intravenous antibiotics. The rate of postoperative wound infection is determined by the intraoperative wound contamination. Rates of infection vary from <5% in simple appendicitis to 20% in cases with perforation and gangrene. The use of perioperative antibiotics has been shown to decrease the rates of post-operative wound infections Third-generation cephalosporins are preferred – a group of broad-spectrum antibiotics, e.g. cefotaxime, ceftazidime, ceftriaxone and moxalactam. However, the antibiotic combination of metronidazole and gentamicin still appears to be in common use. For non-perforated appendicitis, no further antibiotics are required. If the appendix is perforated, antibiotics should be continued until the patient's temperature and WBC count have normalized or continued for a fixed course (Humes and Simpson 2006; Nadler and Gaines 2008).

- Ceftriaxone. *Dose:* 50–100 mg per kilogram of body weight per day (mg/kg per day) once only (e.g. preoperatively) or 1 to 2 times daily for 7–14 days.
- Metronidazole (Flagyl) is used in combination with an aminoglycoside (e.g. Gentamicin), giving broad gram-negative and anaerobic coverage. It appears to be absorbed into cells; intermediate metabolized compounds bind DNA and inhibit protein synthesis, causing cell death. *Dose:* 15–30 mg/kg/d IV divided bd/td for 7 d, or 40 mg/kg PO once; not to exceed 2 g/d.
- Gentamicin (Gentacidin, Garamycin) is an aminoglycoside antibiotic for gram-negative coverage. It is generally used in combination with an agent against gram-positive organisms and one against anaerobes. May be given intravenously or intramuscularly. *Dose:* 15–30 mg/kg/d IV divided bd/td for 7 days, or 40 mg/kg PO once; not to exceed 2 g/d.

All wounds are susceptible to infection, particularly in vulnerable patients with immunosuppression resulting from concurrent health problems and frailty, and depending on the nature of the wound and the ability of the patient to resist infecting organisms (Santy 2008). Wound infection is a serious problem for patients as it may result in delayed wound healing and delay in general recovery, disruption of wound tensile strength and wound dehiscence (breakdown). Wound infection also increases the risk of sepsis and organ failure and may even lead to death (Stotts 2000). Therefore, although antibiotic therapy has been instituted, regular assessment of the wound site is required.

It is essential that nurses are able to identify wounds that are infected, so ensuring that infection is reported and appropriate treatment can begin promptly.

All wounds will display signs of chronic inflammation when infection is present, although inflammation may manifest in different ways. The clinical features of acute inflammation, often seen in acute wound infection, have been recognized. An inflamed wound will often display a combination of features and may be hot, red, swollen and painful, and may also occasionally discharge pus. These features are frequently referred to as the 'classic' or 'cardinal' signs of infection (Cutting and Harding 1994; Woolf 2000).

The inflammatory response can be described as a 'protective mechanism that aims to neutralize and destroy any toxic agents at the site of injury'. This reaction is part of the body's normal response to tissue damage as well as to microbial attack, and involves changes in small blood vessels, adhesion of white blood cells to the inner lining of the vessels and migration of these cells from the blood vessels into the spaces between the cells to deal with invading bacteria and other organisms (Woolf 2000). In acute wounds, this response should only last a day or so, until further microbial attack is prevented by the proliferation of new cells and the wound is sealed (Hart 2002).

Conclusion

Protecting patients from infection means that all healthcare staff should undertake procedures correctly every time, for every patient, in every healthcare setting. There are clear activities and processes that impact on infection and implementing these along the patient pathway can make all the difference in bringing down infection rates (Department of Health 2008:10).

Because of their young age and the immaturity of their immune systems, children are susceptible to infections. Certain children are particularly at risk of HAIs; among these are neutropenic patients and those in intensive and high dependency care settings with indwelling devices. Other risk factors for HAI, such as close physical contact with healthcare workers or stay in environments where antibiotic-resistant organisms are endemic, are common to adult and paediatric patients (Posfay-Barbe *et al.* 2008). However, there must be a combination of factors which allow infection to take hold: the susceptible host, a causative agent, a reservoir, portal of exit, a mode of infection and a portal of entry (Whittaker 2004). The child health nurse has a key role in minimizing the likelihood of an infection taking hold and in being able to identify signs of infection so that early interventions canbe instituted.

Learning activities

- Identify children and young people using your service who may be immunocompromised.
- Find out you local policy for the management of children and young people requiring protective isolation.
- Tunnelled central vascular catheters are commonly used in immunocompromised patients. Find out your local policy for the care and management of such devices.
- Consider the psychological interventions for children and young people who are in isolation. How would you explain or support the following:
  1. isolation procedures and rationales including permitted visiting patterns;
  2. the possible feelings of the child and young person about isolation procedures;
  3. find out the existing coping mechanisms of the child and young person.

References and further reading

Alothman A (2005) Infection control and the immunocompromised host. *Saudi Journal of Kidney Diseases and Transplantation* **16**: 547–555.

Boon NA, Colledge NR, Walker BR, Hunter JAA (eds) (2006) *Davidson's Principles and Practice of Medicine*, 20th Edition. Churchill Livingstone/Elsevier, London.

Callaghan N (2002) Pre-operative fasting. *Nursing Standard* **16**(36): 33–37.

Cohen, MZ, Ley C, Tarzian AJ (2001) Isolation in blood and marrow transplantation. *Western Journal of Nursing Research* **23**(6): 592–609.

Cutting KF, Harding KG (1994) Criteria for identifying wound infection. *Journal of Wound Care* **3**(4): 198–201.

Davies E.G., Elliman DAC, Hart CA, Nicoll A, Rudd PT (2001) *Manual of Childhood Infections*, 2nd Edition. WB Saunders/Royal College of Paediatrics and Child Health, London.

Department of Health (2004) Winning Ways: Working together to reduce Healthcare Associated Infection in England. http://www.dh.gov.uk/en/Publicationsandstatistics/Publications/PublicationsPolicyAnd Guidance/DH_4064682 (accessed 26 July 2008).

Department of Health (2008) Clean, Safe Care – reducing infections and saving lives. www.dh.gov.uk/en/Publicationsandstatistics/Publications/ (accessed 26 July 2008).

Dix K (2005) Clinical Update: Infection Control Practices for the Immuno-compromised Patient Population Infection Control Today. http://www.infectioncontroltoday.com/articles/5c1clinical.html# (accessed 13 February 2009).

Goronzy JJ, Weyand CM (2009) In Lee Goldman L, Shojania K, Shah S (2009) *Cecil's Textbook of Medicine online*. Elsevier. http://textbook.cecilmedicine.com/ (accessed 06 June 2009).

Griffin GE, Sissons JGP, Chiodini PL, Mitchell DM (1999) In Haslett C, Chilvers ER, Hunter JAA, Boon NA (eds) *Davidson's Principles and Practice of Medicine*, 19th Edition. Churchill Livingstone, London.

Griffin J, Arif S, Mufti A (2003) *Crash Course: Immunology and Haematology*, 2nd Edition. Mosby, St Louis, MO, and London.

Grodner M, Long S, DeYoung S (2000) *Foundations and Clinical Applications of Nutrition: a nursing approach*, 2nd Edition. Mosby, St Louis, MO.

Hart J (2002) Inflammation. 1: its role in the healing of acute wounds. *Journal of Wound Care* **11**(6): 205–209.

Hoffbrand AV, Moss P, Petit JE (2006) *Essential Haematology*, 5th Edition. Wiley Blackwell, London.

Humes DJ, Simpson J (2006) Acute appendicitis. *British Medical Journal* **333**: 530–534.

Langton H (2000) *The Child with Cancer*. Bailliere Tindall, London.

Nadler EP, Gaines BA (2008) The Surgical Infection Society guidelines on anti-microbial therapy for children with appendicitis. *Surgical Infections* **9**(1): 75–83.

National Institute for Clinical Excellence (2005) Infection Control: Prevention of healthcare-associated infections in primary and community care. http://www.nice.org.uk/nicemedia/pdf/Infection_control_fullguideline.pdf (accessed 13 January 2009).

Oni L, Dick M, Smalling B; Walters J (2006) *Care and Management of Your Child with Sickle Cell Disease*, 2nd Edition. Department of Health, London.

Phillips B, Selwood K, Lane SM, Skinner R, Gibson F and Chisholm JC (2007) Variation in policies for the management of febrile neutropenia in United Kingdom Children's Cancer Study Group centres. *Archives of Disease in Childhood* **92**: 495–498.

Posfay-Barbe KM, Zerr DM, Pittet D (2008) Infection control in paediatrics. *Lancet Infectious Diseases* **8**: 19–31.

Provan D, Baglin T, Singer CG, Lilleyman JS (2004) *Oxford Handbook of Clinical Haematology*, 2nd Edition. Oxford University Press: Oxford.

Purssell E (2004) Childhood immunology. In Neil S (ed.) *The Biology of Child Health*. Palgrave Macmillan, Basingstoke.

Randall D (2004) Development of the immune system and immunity. In Chamley CA, Carson P, Randall D, Sandwell M (2005) (eds) *Developmental Anatomy and Physiology of Children: a practical approach*. Elsevier/Churchill Livingstone, London.

Santy J (2008) Recognising infection in wounds. *Nursing Standard* **23**(7): 53–60.

Serjeant G, Serjeant B (2001) *Sickle Cell Disease*, 3rd Edition. Oxford Medical Publications, Oxford.

Southgate L, Locke C, Heard S, Wood M (1997) *Infection*. Oxford University Press, Oxford.

Stotts N (2000) Wound infection: diagnosis and management. In Bryant R (ed.) *Acute and Chronic Wounds: nursing management*, 2nd Edition. Mosby, St Louis, MO: 179–188.

Todd WTA, Sundar S, Lockwood DNJ (2006) Principles of infectious disease. In Boon NA, Colledge NR, Walker BR, Hunter JAA (eds) *Davidson's Principles and Practice of Medicine*, 20th Edition. Churchill Livingstone/Elsevier, Edinburgh.

Treacher DF, Grant IS (2006) Critical care and emergency medicine. In Boon NA, Colledge NR, Walker BR, Hunter JAA (Eds) *Davidson's Principles and Practice of Medicine*, 20th Edition. Churchill Livingstone/Elsevier, London.

Whittaker N (2004) *Disorders and Interventions*. Palgrave Macmillan, Basingstoke.

Woolf N (2000) *Cell, Tissue and Disease: the basis of pathology*, 3rd Edition. WB Saunders, Edinburgh.

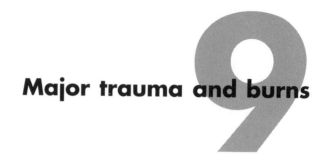

Major trauma and burns

Sheena Carson

Learning outcomes

- To develop an understanding of the assessment processes involved for children who have suffered major trauma or burns
- To develop an understanding of the interventions required for children who have suffered major trauma or burns

Introduction

The aim of this chapter is to consider the assessment and management process of a child presenting with major traumatic injuries or burns using a structured approach, demonstrating the importance of a thorough and accurate assessment to ensure safe and appropriate management. Specific complications associated with these injuries will also be included in the discussion, with relevant evidence utilized throughout to present current recommended practice to manage such complex situations. The identification of a child being abused or at risk will also be addressed, with a specific focus on the child presenting with a non-accidental injury. Scenarios are utilized to consolidate learning.

Trauma

The term 'trauma' is used generally to describe injuries caused by external forces through accidents, acts of violence, or through self harm. Frazer (2007) provides a simple and instructive definition of major trauma as being a 'life- or limb-threatening injury'. Trauma is the most common cause of death in childhood, with road traffic accidents accounting for approximately 80% of injuries. Transport statistics for Great Britain (Department for Transport 2008) stated that, in 2007, 3090 children were killed or seriously injured on the roads, 121 of whom died. Although a significant figure, this is actually 28% fewer than in 2006, and is the lowest ever recorded figure. Through a combination of risk assessment, education and public awareness, improvements are clearly being achieved, making the government's casualty reduction target set in 2000 to reduce by 50% the number of children killed or seriously injured on the roads within 10 years now perhaps more realistic.

While the best cure for trauma still remains prevention, a strong multidisciplinary approach by experienced decision-makers is essential in effective assessment and management of the critically injured child, as failure may have a detrimental effect on mortality and morbidity. Baird *et al.* (2004) suggest that many deaths from trauma that occur after arrival in hospital are preventable, and may occur as a result of missed diagnosis, hypoxia, uncontrolled haemorrhage, or a delay in surgical intervention. More specifically Spahn *et al.* (2007) state that uncontrolled bleeding contributes to approximately 30–40% of trauma-related deaths, highlighting the necessity for early detection followed by prompt intervention to minimize blood loss, restore tissue perfusion, and ultimately restore stability of the child's haemodynamic status. In order to detect potentially life-threatening conditions, a systematic approach must be adopted to assess and manage a critically injured child. The most widely utilized system is the Advanced Paediatric Life Support model (APLS) (Advanced Life Support Group 2005), which prioritizes the assessment and management of each body system. This systematic approach will be adopted for the purpose of this chapter.

Airway with cervical spine control

In all traumatic presentations, a primary survey is commenced with an assessment of the airway, undertaking a *look*, *listen* and *feel* approach with cervical spine control, unless the mechanism of injury clearly rules out the potential for cervical injury. It is of no benefit to the child to proceed onto the assessment of breathing or circulation without first establishing a patent airway, which may potentially be compromised by materials such as blood or vomit, or may be occluded by the tongue. A jaw thrust manoeuvre should be applied to open the airway in a child with suspected cervical spinal injury to prevent further injury, suction can be used to remove foreign material although should be undertaken with caution in the child with a suspected significant head injury as this can cause an elevation in intracranial pressure, and an oro/nasopharyngeal airway can be inserted if the airway is not being maintained.

Breathing with ventilatory support

The assessment moves on to breathing with ventilatory support and it is important to consider that, although a patent airway may have been established, breathing may still not be adequate. If at any time breathing is deemed insufficient, for instance if hypoxaemia or hypercarbia are present, if the child is hyperventilating, or if irregular respirations are evident, then intubation must be considered (National Institute for Clinical Excellence 2007). The aim is to ensure adequate ventilation and oxygenation to prevent the development of complications associated with hypoxia, such as secondary brain injury. In order to identify potential complications associated with respiratory compromise, certain aspects of breathing must be assessed such as the effort required to breathe, the efficacy of these breaths, and the effects on other physiological systems. To aid oxygenation 15 litres of oxygen should be administered via a mask with a reservoir bag.

Careful examination of breathing is required to detect potential life-threatening conditions of the chest which may be present in the child presenting with a traumatic injury, such as:

- airway obstruction
- tension pneumothorax
- open pneumothorax
- massive haemothorax
- flail chest
- cardiac tamponade.

Davies (2002) suggests that chest trauma be divided into two categories: penetrating and blunt. Penetrating refers to when the chest cavity is pierced, blunt trauma where the chest has been compressed or crushed. An important factor to consider is that the degree of external trauma may not fully predict the potential for severe internal injuries, in particular cardiac and vascular injuries. Therefore an accurate account, if available, of the mechanism of injury will aid this assessment process considerably and highlight the potential for the presence of significant injury.

Circulation with haemorrhage control

Once effective ventilation has been established, circulation with haemorrhage control can be assessed. Blunt abdominal trauma is a leading cause of morbidity and mortality among all age groups. The most common cause of blunt abdominal trauma is motor vehicle accidents including those involving pedestrians. Other common aetiologies include falls and industrial or recreational accidents. The liver and spleen seem to be the most frequently injured organs, followed by the small and large intestines.

Both blunt and penetrating injuries have the potential to cause significant bleeding, which in turn can result in a reduction in circulating blood volume, referred to as hypovolaemia, which if not detected and treated promptly can lead to hypovolaemic shock. Early detection of hypovolaemia is essential in preventing potential organ death which results from inadequate perfusion and oxygenation of tissues. The five main sites for potential severe bleeding are the chest, peritoneum, retroperitoneum, pelvis and long bones. The source of bleeding may be obvious on initial assessment, as in penetrating trauma, and obvious bleeding may be managed by applying direct pressure as soon as the patient arrives if appropriate, but should not take priority over the systematic approach described.

Blunt trauma may not be so obvious, so a thorough examination is necessary to determine the presence of external signs of injury such as distention, discoloration, tenderness and deformities. Instability of the lower thoracic cage indicates the potential for splenic or hepatic injuries associated with lower rib injuries.

Pelvic instability indicates the potential for pelvic and retroperitoneal haematoma. Signs of peritonitis such as involuntary guarding, percussion tenderness, or rigidity soon after an injury suggest leakage of intestinal content. Spahn et al. (2007) highlight that traffic accidents are the leading cause of pelvic injury, with an unstable pelvic fracture well documented as being a potential cause of massive haemorrhage. This is echoed by Geeraerts et al. (2007), who state that early evaluation of the severity of the haemodynamically unstable patient should be undertaken as a priority as there is immediate risk to life from haemorrhagic shock. In order to detect ineffective circulatory status, a rapid assessment of heart rate and rhythm, pulse volume and peripheral perfusion should be undertaken. Blood pressure should also be obtained, and the presence of an abnormal respiratory rate and altered mental state considered in the presence of circulatory compromise, as this is an indicator of the effect of shock on other organ systems.

Effective management of a child with circulatory compromise leads with the establishment of vascular access as soon as possible. Peripheral veins are preferred, but in the presence of circulatory insufficiency this option may not be possible due to peripheral vasoconstriction. The cannulation of a central vein is recommended as this allows large volumes of fluid to be administered quickly, which is essential in the presence of hypovolaemic shock. Percutaneous central venous line insertion has replaced peripheral venous cutdown as the initial mode of short-term venous access in children, as cutdown procedures can be time consuming. Central venous cannulation, other than by the femoral route, is hazardous in children and should only be attempted by an experienced practitioner. In very urgent situations the intraosseous route into the tibia is a widely accepted procedure for effective and immediate fluid administration.

Fluid replacement therapy attempts to increase circulatory blood volume and return blood pressure back towards normal parameters which will ensure that the perfusion of vital organs is maintained, thus reversing the effects of hypovolaemia. The type of fluid used continues to be an interesting topic for discussion. The National Institute for Clinical Excellence (2004) identified 10 systematic reviews which compared different intravenous fluid types used for general fluid resuscitation. On the whole there was a potential trend towards crystalloids being more effective than colloids, whereas a recent Cochrane review showed no difference in mortality between those receiving colloids and crystalloids (Roberts *et al.* 2004). In adults, vigorous fluid resuscitation in trauma is not recommended as there is potential to dislodge clot formation in the presence of uncontrolled haemorrhage by raising the blood pressure rapidly. As there are limited studies on the management of fluid resuscitation in paediatric trauma patients, similar guidelines are recommended with fluid boluses of 10 ml/kg with regular reassessment.

Disability with prevention of secondary insult

Once circulating blood volume has been adequately restored and any major haemorrhage controlled, disability and neurological status should be assessed. The potential for a significant head injury in the child presenting following traumatic injury must always be considered during the assessment and management process. The importance of a comprehensive neurological assessment is to provide a baseline and identify the child's normal parameters, to identify the presence and effects of neurological dysfunction, to detect life-threatening situations such as raised intracranial pressure, and to identify changes in condition through continual assessment.

An initial and rapid assessment of consciousness level can be performed using the widely recognized mnemonic scale AVPU, which considers best eye-opening response to stimulus:

- A – Alert
- V – responds to Verbal stimulus
- P – responds to Painful stimulus
- U – Unresponsive.

This scale is only used in the initial stages of the neurological assessment, but can aid in promptly identifying those children with significantly reduced conscious levels, but must be followed up by a more comprehensive assessment as soon as possible. The most widely utilized neurological assessment tool still remains the Glasgow coma scale (GCS); however, the limitations of this tool must be considered when assessing young children or children with physical or learning impairments, therefore adapted scales are available and recommended for use in paediatrics. A decreased level of consciousness may be as a result of several possibilities such as hypoxia, central nervous system injury, drug or alcohol overdose, or hypoglycaemia, which all must be considered, with intubation recommended if the GCS score is below 8 (National Institute for Clinical Excellence 2007). Assessment of pupil size, equality and reaction to light should also be undertaken to detect significant events, such as raised intracranial pressure and compression of cranial nerves II and III.

Exposure with temperature control

Once satisfied with the neurological status, the assessment enters the final stage of exposure: environmental control. Here a top-to-toe survey takes place, considering all other injures, while ensuring hypothermia does not occur. At this stage pain management must be addressed as this will aid compliance during the assessment process, but more significantly, if a head injury is suspected, uncontrolled pain can result in raised intracranial pressure. A balance between pain control and sedation needs to be established to ensure accurate continued assessment, which can be achieved through titration of intravenous morphine 0.1 mg/kg.

Case study 1: 9-year-old who has been involved in a road traffic accident

A 9-year-old boy has been hit by a car while cycling to school. On presentation he is alert and orientated. He is complaining of pain on the right side of his abdomen where there is evident bruising, his right arm and right leg. His heart rate is 140 and his respiratory rate is 35. He is pale and quiet.

Management

The APLS approach should be utilized, commencing with assessment of the boy's airway with cervical spinal immobilization. As he is alert, it can be quickly established that he has a patent airway.

There is a potential for chest trauma due to the mechanism of injury, so an accurate assessment of breathing should be undertaken to identify any traumatic injuries. He is orientated, therefore hypoxia is not an issue at this point but his increased respiratory rate may be due to pain or anxiety, which should be addressed.

His increased heart rate may be a compensatory mechanism to deal with a reduction of circulating volume as a result of internal trauma, which must be considered as he has pain and bruising in the right side of his abdomen, and the mechanism of injury is significant. Early identification and management of circulatory insufficiency will prevent the occurrence of hypovolaemic shock.

As he is alert and orientated, his neurological status is satisfactory at this stage, but will require close monitoring to detect any potential changes which may still occur up to 6 hours after injury.

Assessment of other injuries will detect bleeding from long bones and neurovascular compromise as a result of displaced fractures.

Burns

According to the European Child Safety Alliance (2006), burns and scalds are the fifth leading cause of death of children in the European Union, with over 20 child deaths each year in the United Kingdom as the result of scald injuries. The severity of a burn injury is assessed by the percentage of total body surface involved; with Hettiaratchy and Papini (2004) defining a major burn as covering 25% or more of total body surface area. The aetiology of the burn and the duration of contact with the thermal agent will aid in determining the extent of the injury, therefore history plays a large part in the assessment process. In general the more intense the heat and the longer the duration of contact the deeper the burn injury. Electrical injuries can be deceiving as the extent of tissue damage may be minimal externally, despite more significant internal injuries.

Airway with cervical spine control

As with a traumatic presentation, the primary survey of a child with a burn injury will remain the same beginning with airway, considering cervical spinal control in the absence of a history of the mechanism of injury. With inhalation injuries there is a potential for laryngeal oedema developing several hours after presentation and initial fluid management, so frequent reassessment is essential.

Breathing with ventilatory support

As before, once satisfied that a patent airway is present, the systematic assessment process continues to assess breathing. Respiratory compromise can exist in burn victims as a result of full-thickness circumferential burns to the chest, blast injuries which can cause tension pneumothorax or alveolar trauma, smoke inhalation resulting in inflammation and bronchospasm, and hypoxia as a result of carboxyhaemoglobin. Inhalation of carbon monoxide induces production of carboxyhaemoglobin, which in turn can result in cellular hypoxia. The presence of stridor, hoarse voice, wheeze, or soot in the nose, mouth or sputum clinically indicates smoke inhalation. In the presence of these symptoms or suspicion of smoke inhalation, blood carboxyhaemoglobin should be measured as in these cases pulse oximeters are an unreliable method of identifying hypoxia. Levels of 5–20% can be treated with oxygen, but levels over 20% require a more aggressive approach in a hyperbaric oxygen chamber. As with trauma, adequate oxygenation and ventilation remains the priority, so 100% oxygen should be administered via a mask and a reservoir bag. If respiratory compromise is evident, then this should be dealt with promptly before continuing with the assessment.

Circulation

Once the burn reaches 30% of the total body surface area, the child is at risk of systemic hypotension and organ hypoperfusion as a result of increased capillary permeability, which in turn leads to a loss of fluid into the interstitial compartment and decreased myocardial contractility. Hypermetabolism may also occur, as demonstrated by Jeschke *et al.* (2007) who compared four different burn sizes and found that hypermetabolism occurred in partnership with an increase in burn size. Intravenous access is a priority with two large-bore cannulae sited in unburned skin where possible. Rapid fluid shift and drying out of eschar can result in compromised circulation, with circumferential burns to limbs acting as a tourniquet, potentially compromising blood flow to the limb, so must be managed with an escharotomy as a matter of urgency to prevent potential cell death.

Fluid resuscitation is based on the estimation of the burn surface area mentioned earlier, which can be performed using specific charts. The Land and Browder chart is the most widely used within paediatrics, as it is more accurate in assessing children than the 'rule of nines' or palm size (New Zealand Guidelines Group 2007). It divides the body into areas while taking into consideration the varied proportions in children of different ages. The burned areas are drawn on the chart during assessment using different colours to represent partial thickness, where the epidermis and the upper and deeper layers of the dermis are affected, or full thickness involving damage to all skin layers down to the subcutaneous tissues. The areas are then added up to give an accurate total body surface area, on which treatment is then based. Superficial burns involving the epidermis alone are not counted in this calculation.

Initial fluid resuscitation for shock, if indicated, is recommended as crystalloid solution in bolus doses of 20 ml/kg. If the burn injury is 10% of total body surface area or more, the child will require fluids additional to their normal requirements. The additional fluid calculated in millilitres per day is estimated using the Parkland formula (*percentage burn × weight (kg) × 4*), with half of this additional fluid to be given in the first 8 hours following the time of the burn injury.

This formula was first developed in 1968, and is based on the concepts of fluid shifts between compartments following a severe burn found in studies undertaken by Baxter and Shire. Although this remains the mostly widely utilized resuscitation formula in the world, it has recently come under scrutiny as to whether it is the most accurate method of predicting fluid requirements in burn-injured patients (Csontos *et al.* 2007; Klein *et al.* 2007). Alvarado *et al.* (2009) suggest that while significant progress has been made in the resuscitation of severely burned patients, the guidelines and formulae used today remain those introduced more than 40 years ago, suggesting that further research is required to ensure that a full understanding of burn pathophysiology underpins potential changes in future resuscitation techniques.

Accurate monitoring of the cardiovascular state is essential during fluid resuscitation to assess the effectiveness of the intervention. An accurate method of doing this is by monitoring the urine output through catheterization, with an aim to maintain the urine output at 2 ml/kg/h or more.

Disability with prevention of secondary insult

When assessing the child's neurological state, it is important to consider that reduced consciousness levels following burns may be due to hypoxia, head injury or hypovolaemia. As stated earlier, in the absence of an accurate history a significant head injury or other injuries cannot be ruled out, particularly in blast injuries.

Exposure with temperature control

Again a top-to-toe survey is essential to consider all other injures that might have been sustained, while ensuring hypothermia does not occur as burned children have the potential to lose heat rapidly through convection and evaporation. Relieving pain must be seen as a priority and, as in trauma, intravenous morphine 0.1 mg/kg should be administered. Entonox is often underutilized in emergency situations and can be an effective pain-relieving intervention for the appropriately aged child during the initial stages until intravenous access has been established and further analgesia organized. The intramuscular route is not recommended in burn injuries as absorption is unreliable.

Referral/Transfer

It must be recognized when a child with a burn injury requires specialist care; therefore clear criteria should be in place to guide practitioners. These criteria tend to be individual to each hospital trust, but in general should include:

- 10% partial- and/or full-thickness burns;
- 5% full-thickness burns;
- Burns to special areas: face, mouth, hands and feet can result in severe functional loss due to scarring;
- Perineal burns: prone to infection and difficult to manage;
- Circumferential burns;
- Significant inhalation burn;
- Chemical, radiation or high voltage electrical burns: depth of the burn usually greater than apparent and complications of cardiac arrhythmias (Advanced Life Support Group 2005).

Ansermino and Hemsley (2004) state that up to 75% of mortality in burns patients following the initial resuscitation phase is related to infection, as the wound site is the perfect environment for bacterial growth; therefore, while awaiting transfer or further management of the injury, the burn should be protected. Clingfilm is an ideal dressing as it protects the wound while still allowing visualization of the injury, thus avoiding repeated removal of dressings which can be extremely painful and distressing for the child.

Safeguarding

As with any other presentation, the suspicion of non-accidental injury must not be overlooked in the trauma or burn victim. Accurate history taking can aid in detecting potential cause for concern, such as a delay in presentation, inconsistencies in the history, or a discrepancy between the history given and the injury itself. Any type of fracture may be seen in the child being abused, but there are several features specifically associated with non-accidental injury. These include fractures in a child under 2 years of age without a significant history, multiple fractures in varied stages of healing, spiral fractures of long bones, rib fractures and skull fractures. Other significant signs include perioral injuries, retinal haemorrhages and ruptured internal organs without a history of major trauma, and perianal or genital injury. In the child presenting with a burn or scald, signs for concern include such things as the detection of obvious patterns to the burn such as burns caused by cigarettes or an iron, an absence of splash marks in scald injuries, signs of restraint on upper limbs, or an obvious tidal pattern from being forcibly put into a bath.

Hettiartchy and Dziewulski (2004) estimate that around 3–10% of paediatric burn injuries are due to non-accidental injury, with children younger than 3 years of age most commonly affected. Differentiating between an intentional and non-intentional burn or scald is an extremely challenging situation. Maguire *et al.* (2008) conducted a systematic review with the aim of identifying distinguishing features of intentional and unintentional scalds. A total of 26 observational and retrospective studies were included, representing 587 children, 183 of whom sustained intentional scalds. Forced immersion scald injuries were consistently described as the most common mechanism of intentional injury, with hot tap water the predominant thermal agent. The commonest affected areas were bilateral lower extremities, buttocks and perineal area; however, upper extremity areas may also be affected, with facial immersion more rare. In contrast, unintentional accidental scalds tended to be as a result of spills where the child pulled a container of hot liquid off a table or cooker. Accidental hot water immersion scalds were uncommon.

Safeguarding children is a shared responsibility, with early detection of abuse paramount. The welfare of the child is literally in the hands of the practitioner; therefore the potential for non-accidental injury in the child presenting with traumatic injuries or burns should always remain at the forefront of any assessment. According to the government-issued national guideline *Working Together to Safeguard Children* (Department for Education and Skills 2006), all health professionals have a duty to protect children, with an emphasis on interagency communication to ensure a collaborative approach to the promotion of children's welfare, and prevent them from suffering harm. According to the latest World Health Organization figures, there has been a major reduction in the number of violence-related deaths in children in England and Wales since the 1970s, perhaps demonstrating some effective, steady progress in early assessment and intervention strategies, thus protecting more children from the extreme end of abuse.

Case study 2: 2-year-old with burns

A 2-year-old has presented with burn injuries to his lower legs. His mother states that she was running a bath for the child last night and when she left the room for a minute the child fell into the bath. She put him to bed after, but decided to come to hospital today as the marks on his legs were still there. On examination the child is very distressed. Burns have been sustained to both feet up to mid-calf level. No splash marks are evident, and no other injuries are obvious.

Management

A systematic approach should be utilized to accurately assess the child.

Accurate assessment and documentation of the depth of the injuries and calculation of the total surface body area affected will determine the treatment options, i.e. whether fluid resuscitation is required, or transfer to specialist treatment unit as burns are to the feet.

Non-accidental injury should be suspected in this situation as the mechanism of injury does not reflect the injuries sustained, along with a delay in presentation and a possible history of a lack of supervision if the history is to be believed.

This child may have suffered significant harm, so a full investigation will be required; ensuring the safety of the child remains central throughout the process.

Conclusion

Caring for a child and their family following a traumatic event can be extremely challenging for the less confident or less experienced practitioner. This chapter has highlighted that by following a structured systematic approach, the prioritization and management of the most significant injuries is ensured, thus limiting the potential for misdiagnosis or mismanagement. In the absence of a clear history, an accurate assessment is essential in detecting potential life-threatening complications, so should therefore be undertaken by an experienced practitioner with the relevant knowledge, skills and ability to ensure the best possible outcome for the child. The potential for deterioration at any stage should never be underestimated; therefore assessment must be considered as a continual process incorporated into the overall management of the child. The psychological needs of both the child and their family should not be overlooked during this process, as suffering a major traumatic injury or burn can be an extremely distressing experience. Continuous reassurance and effective communication can aid in reducing levels of anxiety, resulting in a more compliant child, which in turn will ensure a more positive experience for all involved.

Learning activities

- Reflect upon a child you have cared for who has suffered a traumatic injury. How did you discuss the mechanism of the injury with the child and family? What features would lead you to consider the possibility of non-accidental injury?
- Reflect upon a child who has suffered a burn. How do you think their body image may be affected by the injury?
- What factors are important when choosing wound dressings to use on bums? Look at the dressings that are available in your clinical area and decide if they are appropriate.

References and further reading

Advanced Life Support Group (2005) *Advanced Paediatric Life Support: the practical approach*, 4th Edition. Blackwell Publishing, Oxford.

Alvarado R, Chung K, Cancio L, Wolf S (2009) Burn resuscitation. *Burns* **35**(1): 4–14.

Ansermino M, Hemsley C (2004) ABC of burns: intensive care management and control of infection. *British Medical Journal* **329**: 220–223.

Baird C, Kernohan G, Coates V (2004) Outcomes of advanced trauma life support training: questioning the role of observer. *Accident and Emergency Nursing* **12**(3): 131–135.

Clinical Knowledge Summaries (2007) Burns and scalds. http://www.cks.library.nhs.uk/burns_and_scalds (accessed 05 February 2009).

Csontos C, Foldi V, Fischer T, Bogar L (2007) Factors affecting fluid requirement on the first day after severe burn trauma. *ANZ Journal of Surgery* **77**(9): 745–749.

Dale P, Green R, Fellows R (2002) Serious and fatal injuries to infants with discrepant parental explanations: some assessment and case management issues. *Child Abuse Review* **11**: 296–312.

Davies K (2002) Blunt chest trauma: a challenge to accident and emergency nurses. *Accident and Emergency Nursing* **10**(4): 197–204.

Department for Education and Skills (2006) *Working Together to Safeguard Children*. http://www.ecm.gov.uk/workingtogether/ (accessed 05 February 2009).

Department for Transport (2008) *Road casualties Great Britain: 2007*. http://www.dft.gov.uk (accessed 04 February 2009).

European Child Safety Alliance (2006) http://www.childsafetyeurope.org (accessed 05 February 2009).

Frazer A (2007) Major Trauma: assessment prioritization and initial treatment In Evans C, Tippins E (eds) (2007) *The Foundations of Emergency Care*. Open University Press, Maidenhead.

Geeraerts T, Chhor V, Cheisson G, Martin L, Bessoud B, Ozanne A, Duranteau J (2007) Clinical review: initial management of blunt pelvic trauma patients with haemodynamic instability. *Critical Care* **11**: 204.

Haas N (2004) Clinical review: vascular access for fluid infusion in children. *Critical Care* **8**: 478–484.

Hettiaratchy S, Dziewulski P (2004) ABC of burns: pathophysiology and types of burns. *British Medical Journal* **328**: 1427–1429.

Hettiaratchy S, Papini R (2004) ABC of burns: initial management of a major burn: 1. overview. *British Medical Journal* **328**: 1555–1557.

Holland A, Jackson A, Joseph A (2005) Paediatric trauma at an adult trauma centre. *ANZ Journal of Surgery* **75**(10): 878–881.

Jeschke M, Mlcak RP, Finnerty CC, Norbury WB, Gauglitz GG, Kulp GA, Herndon DN (2007) Burn size determines the inflammatory and hypermetabolic response. *Critical Care* **11**: R90.

Klein M, Hayden D, Elson C, Nathens AB, Gamelli RL, Gibran NS *et al.* (2007) The association between fluid administration and outcome following major burn. *Annals of Surgery* **245**(4): 622–628.

Kwan I, Bunn F, Roberts I (2003) Timing and volume of fluid administration for patients with bleeding. *Cochrane Database Systematic Reviews*, CD002245.

Maguire S, Moynihan S, Mann M, Potokar T, Kemp AM (2008) A systematic review of the features that indicate intentional scalds in children. *Burns* **34**(8): 1072–1081.

McCance K, Heuther S (2006) *Pathophysiology: the biologic basis for disease in adults and children*, 5th Edition. Elsevier Mosby, St Louis, MO.

National Institute for Clinical Excellence (2004) Pre-hospital initiation of fluid replacement therapy in trauma. http://www.nice.org.uk (accessed 05 February 2009).

National Institute for Clinical Excellence (2007) Triage, assessment, investigation and early management of head injury in infants, children and adults. http://www.nice.org.uk (accessed 05 February 2009).

New Zealand Guidelines Group (2007) Management of burns and scalds in primary care: evidence-based best practice guideline. http://www.nzgg.org.nz (accessed 05 February 2009).

Pritchard C, Sharples A (2008) 'Violent' deaths of children in England and Wales and the major developed countries 1974–2002: possible evidence of improving child protection? *Child Abuse Review* **17**: 297–312.

Roberts I, Alderson P, Bunn F, Chinnock P, Ker K, Schierhout G (2004) Colloids versus crystalloids for fluid resuscitation in critically ill patients. *Cochrane Database Systematic Reviews*, CD000567.

Spahn D, Cerny V, Coats T, Duranteau J, Fernandez-Mondejar E, Gordini G *et al.* (2007) Management of bleeding following major trauma: a European guideline. *Critical Care* **11**: 414.

Spencer D (2002) Paediatric trauma: when is it not an accident? *Accident and Emergency Nursing* **10**: 143–148.

Technology-dependent children and complex care

10

Paula Kelly and Deborah Lynn

Learning outcomes

- To understand what is meant by complex care and technology-dependent
- To demonstrate knowledge of the clinical and psychosocial issues for children with complex care needs and their families in hospital and in the transition from hospital to home
- To have an understanding of the challenges of delivering paediatric palliative care for children with high dependency needs

Introduction

This chapter will focus on the care of children who have ongoing high dependency needs, drawing on clinical case studies and empirical research to illustrate the key factors. It differs from the previous chapters in the text in that it crosses the boundaries of a single system or disease pathology and focuses on the shared principles of nursing care that children and families require. In addition it reflects the location of care outside the inpatient care setting but requiring the support and resources that are predominantly located not merely in patient settings overall but particularly within the more specialist of those services. This ongoing need for care that crosses boundaries is a key challenge to providers in meeting the needs of children and families.

The chapter commences with an examination of the concepts of technology-dependent and complex care as applied to the nursing care of children and families. Discussion focuses on an approach to assessment and intervention that recognizes the limitations that a rigid application of these terms may imply for service delivery. This section is required to highlight for practitioners the challenges in operational policy guidance for this group of children and provides a contextual setting for the case studies and care themes that follow. The following section aims to examine high dependency in transition, looking at the organizational issues in transferring children's care from an acute inpatient setting to home. The challenges of meeting high dependency needs in the home setting are then explored. Finally, the implications of palliative care for children with high dependency care requirements are considered, providing an example that identifies the need for several service sectors to provide rapid response in a coordinated manner. The chapter concludes with an identification of the practice and research challenges for practitioners to develop high-quality care packages to meet the need of current and future children and families requiring high dependency care in the long term.

Contextualizing the care group

Defining concepts – In the latter half of the twentieth century clinicians began to document and investigate the care needs of a group of children whom they termed technology-dependent (Wagner *et al.* 1988). They described these children as those

> 'Who need both a medical device to compensate for the loss of a vital body function and substantial and ongoing nursing care to avert death or further disability' (p. 3).

The group included children who required mechanical ventilation, oxygen therapy, enteral feeding and intravenous therapy. As Kirk and Glendinning (2004) argue, the children not only depended on a wide range of technologies (including multiple technologies for some children) but could also vary according to the intensity of their nursing care requirements. In addition their prognosis could be life limiting or life threatening and they could experience cognitive, developmental and/or physical disability alongside their technology dependence.

This small but expanding heterogeneous group of children drew attention in part because of their prolonged hospitalization beyond a time when they were thought to be benefiting from care in this setting (Noyes 2002). The drive to reduce healthcare costs and provide a more optimum long-term care environment resulted in exploring the potential for discharge and home care. The availability of more portable technology and a shift in the expectations on where and by whom 'technological' care could be delivered resulted in the drive to facilitate care in the home setting for technology-dependent children.

Despite some evidence suggesting that this is an expanding group of children, there is little robust data on the precise numbers of children that fall under this umbrella term; Graham *et al.* (2008) suggest 1 per 1000 children in the United States. In the United Kingdom, Glendinning *et al.* (2001) used a range of data sources to estimate the numbers of children requiring this type of care. Their figure of 6000, although thought to underestimate the actual numbers, is the last published attempt to quantify this group of children, based on UK empirical data. As they and other authors have suggested, both the lack of complete data records and the category itself is problematic and is sometimes replaced by the term 'complex continuing care needs' (Carnevale *et al.* 2008; Muir and Dryden 2000). Others use this term not to denote dependency in the technological sense but to reflect the complexities of children's care needs. Lenton *et al.* (2004) helpfully argue that it refers to those who require care packages that require, health, social and educational services to work together jointly. This definition includes children who are highly dependent on care but are excluded from technology-dependent care, such as children with autism spectrum disorders. This corresponds with the care definitions outlined in the national service framework (Department of Health 2005a). The benefit of this approach is that it guides practitioners towards care needs for children and families rather than a categorization dependent upon diagnosis or the presence of technology.

The Department of Health (2008a) consultation on assessment for continuing healthcare needs has piloted a framework that seeks to standardize the eligibility criteria for children to receive additional packages of health care. Using ten care domains, the assessment process aims to use information to determine levels of need for the child that reflect the complexity, intensity and unpredictability of need and risk associated with maintaining their health. For example, a child with a tracheostomy may have a stable or unpredictable pattern of suction requirements. Although this tool will undoubtedly prove valuable in helping practitioners and commissioners determine eligibility and funding for services, it may not eliminate some of the differences in levels of care that families receive across the country or even within the same commissioning and providing service. In order to achieve this broader objective, debate is required that addresses the levels of support that communities are prepared to commit in order to provide long-term care for children whose health needs may have been expected to be met in the high-technology environments of paediatric intensive care and high dependency units. Practitioners, service providers and commissioners together with children and parents need to question their expectations of parenting roles and if nursing care can ever usefully be seen as a separate entity from child care. When we encourage parents in the hospital setting to participate in their children's care in a technologically focused hospital environment there is an acknowledgement of their knowledge as experts in their child, and their learning of technical nursing and medical skills may facilitate their involvement in care and extend their opportunities for informed decision-making. In addition these activities extend parental responsibilities, possibly leaving these parents to cover nursing breaks in the inpatient environment and to manage with variable levels of support in the community setting.

This review serves to illustrate that this group of children are likely to be heterogeneous (Kirk *et al.* 2005), even in cases where the same technology is required (Noyes and Lewis 2007; Koglmeier *et al.* 2008). Research carried out by Kirk and Glendinning (2004) in the United Kingdom does suggest that both younger children and those with respiratory conditions are highly represented in the cohort. In addition the geographical distribution of children requiring this care in the long term also appears to be uneven (While *et al.* 2004), an important factor when considering service planning and costs to local providers. As Primary Care Trusts develop their commissioning roles (Thornley 2008), data sets that enable better predictive data on the numbers of local children who might require technology-dependent care may enable local providers to be responsive to any specific local needs, for example where there are high rates of prematurity and very low birthweight babies.

Transition from hospital to home

Case study 1: 5-year-old with Down syndrome and spinal injury

Sayed, aged 5, has Down syndrome; 4 months ago he was involved in a road traffic accident and sustained damage to his spinal cord. He now has a tracheostomy and requires overnight positive pressure ventilation. Following a period of time in the paediatric intensive care unit, he has been nursed on the high dependency unit of the children's hospital. Prior to this he lived at home with two older siblings and his parents. He attended the local school for children with special needs. Sayed's mother and siblings are bilingual and fluent English speakers while his father has limited English language skills.

Management

Planning and executing the discharge home of a child who is dependent on technology is based on the same principles of discharge as any other child and family (Department of Health 2004a) (Box 10.1). In essence it should be smooth and timely; services delivered to families build on the coherent cooperation of multiagency services organized around the needs of families. Meeting these expectations has been demonstrated to be particularly challenging for children who are technology dependent (Noyes and Lewis 2005; Stephens 2005). Box 10.1 proposes a number of activities for consideration and, although each child and family's specific needs will vary, this list provides a useful summary.

Jardine and Wallis (1998), on behalf of the UK Long-Term Ventilation Working Party, define ventilation dependence as continuing to require mechanical ventilation, three months after initiation in the context of medical stability.

Medical stability may be defined differentially in technology-dependent children; in broad terms it is taken to mean being able to maintain system functionality to an acceptable level, maintaining a healthy state, and a state that enables physical, psychological and social development within the child's potential. In Sayed's case medical stability related to his being able to maintain adequate respiratory function during the day,

---

Box 10.1 **Discharge planning process**

- Establish medical stability
- Discussion with child and family on implications of home management and prolonged hospitalization
- Needs assessment
- Identification of key worker
- Discharge proposal by case manager
- Multidisciplinary planning meeting
- Funding confirmed
- Identification of home support services (recruitment and selection)
- Purchase and installation of home-based equipment/ adaptations
- Training
- Moving home
- Ongoing support including respite and management of acute episodes

without ventilation support, and overnight having a stable rate and ventilation pressures. This was evaluated through a comprehensive assessment of respiratory function including monitoring his oxygen saturations through non-invasive pulse oximetry overnight and maintaining this at 95% or above. His respiratory rate and effort, and heart rate were within his normal limits. Other observations included being alert to other signs of declining respiratory function, such as requiring more frequent suction, changes in the nature of secretions, increased cough, the presence of wheeze, changes in concentration and levels of consciousness.

Sayed's family lived in an area where there was an established community children's nursing service (Eaton 2001), although the service had no experience at that time of managing a ventilator-dependent child (Cejer 2007). Early engagement with this service was essential to establish key worker responsibilities, and to engage with the commissioning authorities who would provide the financial resources to support the care package required by Sayed and his family to enable discharge (Noyes *et al.* 2006). One of the senior nurses from the service worked jointly with a member of the hospital outreach service to carry out a needs assessment. This assessment used the common assessment framework as a template to ensure that all aspects of Sayed's health and well-being were considered (Department of Health 2000). The National Service Framework includes an exemplar on long-term ventilation (Department of Health 2005b) that practitioners can now use as guidance in planning and commissioning appropriate service provision. This assessment process included visits to the family home, identifying and incorporating other professionals such as occupational therapists to advise and cost home adaptations, and working with a bilingual health advocate to ensure that Sayed's father was able to participate fully in the assessment process. This resource-intensive joint approach by the community and hospital services facilitated joint engagement in the discharge process, leading to shared knowledge and responsibility. Sayed's family were reassured that the hospital service were still actively committed to his care, and their professional working relationship with the 'new' community team enabled a transition of trust for the family.

An example of how this worked in practice was the joint development of the family-held records and the care pathway to use at home to guide responses to changes in care needs and any deterioration. It was important that these documents drew on the clinical expertise of the high dependency hospital services and the community nurses' knowledge of care issues in the home setting. Hospital environments are designed to accommodate equipment and enable professionals to carry out their roles; home environments are geared towards a different purpose. In Sayed's case prolonged hospitalization occurred as adaptations could not be made to his family's home and they required rehousing by the local authority. This illustrates the need not only for multi-agency health work in planning successful discharge but to include other agencies as an early stage.

The confirmation of funding for a care package to support the purchase and maintenance costs of equipment (for example portable ventilators, suction catheters, tracheostomy tubes, suction machines) and the salary costs for nurses and carers is cited as a frequent source of delay in children being transferred to home care (Noyes 2002; While *et al.* 2004). In this case effective arrangements for joint local commissioning between health and social care (Department for Education and Skills/Department of Health 2006a) alongside a proactive Primary Care Trust children's commissioner resulted in a prompt decision in response to the assessments and funding requests submitted by the team leader of the local community children's nursing team, who had taken on the role of key worker for Sayed and his family. The package of care approved included ten hours of care overnight seven nights a week, in recognition of Sayed's vulnerability during ventilation, and two hours of care five days a week, at a time to be agreed with the family. This care was to be provided by healthcare support workers trained and supervised by a registered children's nurse for which the package contributed 0.2 of a band 6 salary to be part of the community children's nursing service. In addition the commissioners agreed to fully fund the equipment outlined in the proposal prepared.

Meeting the education and support needs of Sayed's family and the newly recruited team of carers required joint expertise. During the assessment process Sayed's father reported that, although he felt technically competent in relation to tracheostomy care, his emotional response to carrying out care such as suction that distressed his child had not been accounted for in the training provided. This concern echoes that demonstrated in Kirk *et al.*' s study (2005) in which parents suggested that developing technical competence was the primary focus of training packages provided in hospital settings. This suggests that 'risk' to technology-dependent children is constructed primarily in terms of equipment failure or failure to manage technology by clinical staff. Although this is an important source of 'risk', it fails to acknowledge the social and emotional impact on parents and staff in caring for technology-dependent children outside the intensive care or high dependency inpatient setting.

This section has focused on the complex process of discharge which can be seen as a series of transitions that children, families and staff are required to manage rather than a rigid boundary between care in hospital and care at home. Initial care at home may be interspersed with returns to the hospital as a staged transfer. Some neonatal and transitional care units have provision for parents to 'practise' home care within the hospital environment with minimal staff involvement. Children's hospice services who have played a key role in providing respite care for children with life-limiting conditions can also provide a way of staging discharge for some children who are technology dependent. By providing a package of transitional care they can enable training for families and carers if required in an environment that is more home-like than an acute hospital unit. Their multidisciplinary approach to care can also provide families with a broader network of support services than those available from universal services in their local Primary Care Trust. Whichever model of transfer is adopted, as the following section will illustrate, technology-dependent children require ongoing access to hospital services.

Challenges at home

Case study 2: 18-month-old with short bowel syndrome

David is 18 months and has spent most of his life in hospital; he was born at 34 weeks' gestation, with a very low birthweight. Aged 10 days he developed necrotizing enterocolitis which did not respond to conservative management and he required surgical resection of a considerable portion of his bowel. As a result he has short bowel syndrome and requires parenteral nutrition (PN). David lives at home with his mother who is a lone parent; they have no contact with his father and her extended family live in another part of the country several miles away.

Management

This section examines some of the challenges to families and professionals in the care of technology-dependent children at home, with a focus on monitoring well-being in the home setting, potential burden of care for families and the need for respite.

Research with families who have experienced caring for their technology-dependent child at home suggests that the simple transfer of hospital equipment, routines and practices to the home setting, 'hospital at home', is problematic (Carnevale *et al.* 2006; Heaton *et al.* 2006; Yantzi *et al.* 2006). This can be illustrated by a consideration of the monitoring practices of care in the home setting: there had been a good deal of debate in relation to the use of monitoring equipment for children who are oxygen dependent, suggesting that the use of constant pulse oximetry increases parental anxiety (Murphy 2001), alongside evidence that formal saturation studies can be predictive of life-threatening events in infants receiving oxygen at home (Harrison *et al.* 2006).

In planning David's care at home, the clinical team and his mother agreed that daily weighing, which had been a routine aspect of his hospital care, was of limited benefit. David had been stable on his 18-hour cyclical PN for several months prior to discharge and weekly monitoring of electrolytes was reduced to monthly testing shortly after home discharge. The timing of the blood tests to monitor his electrolytes needed to take into account both the disruption this could cause to the newly established home routines, and also the processes involved in ensuring that results were available to appropriate staff for review. In addition consideration was given to the likely increased risks of catheter-related problems of infection, occlusion and thromboembolism (Ryder 2006; Kakazanov 2008).

Life at home for David and his mother presented additional challenges; as Holden (2001) reported, social isolation for families of children on PN is common. Although David's infusion fluids and pump were compact (being accommodated in a small rucksack), leaving home even for short periods required considerable pre-planning (Yantzi *et al.* 2006). In addition the family had lost the social contact with staff and other families that was available in the hospital setting. The uneven provision and limited availability of respite care services for children with ongoing health problems continues to be well documented (Macdonald and Callery 2004; Heaton *et al.* 2005; Thurgate 2005). Although an overnight carer to minimize sleep disruption for David's mother from infusion alarms during the night (Heaton *et al.* 2006) was part of the initial care package, funding could not be secured for this. David's mother expressed some ambivalence about having another person in her home while she was asleep (Margolan *et al.* 2004). In addition she was concerned that the proposal suggested this would not be a healthcare professional rather a lay carer who would receive additional training (Royal College of Nursing 2008). Indeed, David's mother suggested although the technical skills could be learnt, for a 'stranger' to take on the responsibilities of David's well-being without the foundations of a professional qualification was 'a lot to ask'. The community children's nursing service, who took on the key worker role in David's care, suggested attendance at a local opportunity playgroup for David and his mother, two afternoons a week. This service gave contact with other children and parents and support with David's care. In addition flexible daytime respite at home was slowly developed in conjunction with a local children's charity that also provided transport support to families of children with health problems to enable David's mother to have time at home or outside the home for short breaks. This is one initiative cited by Stanley (2008) as a good practice example of flexible short breaks. Funding is now available, under the umbrella of the *Aiming High for Disabled Children* initiatives (Department of Health 2008b), to increase the opportunities for children with disabilities to have time away from their primary carer and to increase their participation in activities that other children take for granted as part of childhood., This would now be of benefit to David, given that children with complex needs form one of the priority groups for this funding. David's mother also joined an online parental discussion group, making contact with other families of children on parenteral feeding, which she felt decreased her feelings of isolation and dependence on professionals (Green 2007).

Growing up with technology

Case study 3

Stacey is 15 years old and has cystic fibrosis which was diagnosed in early infancy. As a young child she had numerous hospital admissions with chest infections, requiring intensive physiotherapy, intravenous antibiotics and respiratory support. She now requires continuous low-flow oxygen and has required ventilator support on her last two hospital admissions, receiving CPAP via a mask. She has a gastrostomy for overnight feeding and insulin therapy. Stacey lives at home with her parents and three siblings, her eldest sister has recently gone to university and her older brother is applying to do so next year. Her youngest sister is still at primary school.

Management

Although Stacey has had a long and close involvement with hospital services, in particular the cystic fibrosis service at the children's hospital thirty miles from her home, her dependence on technology has been gradually increasing as has her need for high dependency care in the inpatient context. A cystic fibrosis nurse is her key worker, coordinating services in the hospital and the community, providing information and advice to the family, identifying and addressing need and acting as an advocate (Beresford 2005). As Stacey's need for technology support has increased, additional support has been organized in the school setting to enable her continued attendance (Wray 2008). Facilitating this involved her local Diana Community children's nursing service which provides education and training to teaching assistants and other school staff. A care plan was developed jointly with the school nurse, cystic fibrosis nurse specialist and the community children's nursing service to provide the school staff with guidance on how to manage the oxygen delivery in the school setting in a safe manner and how to recognize and respond appropriately to any changes in Stacey's care needs during the school day. As discussed in the previous section, this work involves attention to the care of technology and the physiological implications of reduced respiratory function to be explored in a manner that enables understanding for those without healthcare training. The team made use of training packs and associated carer competencies developed by the complex needs team at Coventry and Warwickshire Primary Care Trust (available from www.act.org.uk/indexphp/teaching-framework. htlm) as a framework and applied the evidence-based materials to meet Stacey's specific needs. In addition the implications of Stacey's need for increasing interventions and her experiences in recent hospital admissions also raised concerns within the school from staff and pupils about Stacey's long-term prognosis. The local service gained consent from Stacey and her family to explore with staff and pupils the emotional impact of her illness, and worked with the clinical psychologist attached to the local children's hospice to facilitate sessions. Recognition of the emotional impact of caring for children with life-limiting conditions is an important consideration for staff when undertaking liaison with community and hospital-based high dependency staff. In Stacey's case there were differences in perceptions around her quality of life between hospital and community nurses that required exploration in order to promote effective joint working.

This work was carried out within a context of considering the planning and implementation of transitioning Stacey's care from children's services to adult services (Department for Education and Skills/Department of Health 2006b?). Some of the organizational issues that planning Stacey's transition highlighted were that although the hospital-based children's services had an end of eligibility marker of age 16, the Diana Community children's service was able to see children at home until the age of 19. The services together with Stacey and her family decided that this differential had some benefits as it enabled a staged transition process (ACT 2007). Stacey chose to begin attending the joint young people and adult cystic fibrosis outpatient clinics after her last admission to intensive care when it was discussed that if she required intensive care treatment in subsequent exacerbations she could be admitted to an adult unit. At the clinic, which was held on alternate dates within adult services, Stacey was able to develop relationships with the adult nursing and medical staff. In the community setting, staff and Stacey met to develop a joint transition pathway that identified the key care needs and the resources that Stacey felt she needed in place to meet these. Stacey wanted to have a stronger voice in making decisions about her care but she felt the need for training in relation to this, joining a group of young people with long-term health conditions who were linked to the Expert Patients programme.

Palliative care

Death in childhood is a rare event even for health professionals working with children with serious illness who are dependent on technology. The following categories of paediatric palliative care may all include children with high dependency needs.

- Conditions for which potentially curative treatment has failed (e.g. malignancy).
- Conditions where intensive treatment may prolong or enhance life, but premature death still occurs (e.g. cystic fibrosis, AIDS).
- Progressive conditions where treatment is almost exclusively pallia-tive but may extend over many years (e.g. neurodegenerative conditions).
- Non-progressive neurological conditions which result in an increased susceptibility to complications and premature death (e.g. severe cerebral palsy).

Towards the end of the last century children with progressive neu-rological conditions overtook children with malignancies as the largest single group for paediatric palliative care services in particular chil-dren's hospices (Horrocks *et al.* 2002; Elston 2003). Technological support as described in this chapter has shifted the time of initiation and dura-tion of paediatric palliative care for children in some diagnostic groups, for example cystic fibrosis. The end of curative treatment and the com-mencement of palliative treatment is realized with less well-defined boundaries, with Liben *et al.* (2008) suggesting that an integrated service approach is required where children and families have contact with palliative care services blended with their ongoing treatment services. The model they present offers considerable potential for shared exper-tise in symptom control management (Willis 2007) and opportunities to consider the ethical and practical questions raised in relation to the withdrawal or maintenance of invasive technological treatment regimes (Parker *et al.* 1999; Bush *et al.* 2005; Gillis 2008). This model also provides an opportunity for staff working in curative-based services to work closely with palliative care services, which may enable more staff to be confident in discussing palliative care with families rather than a situ-ation where staff feel reluctant to address these issues with families, leading to confusion and in some cases lost opportunities for families having more time with their child in a setting of their choice.

Children's palliative care services are increasingly recognizing that palliative care for this group of children presents specific challenges, including bereavement care that recognizes the specialized parenting roles that that been undertaken and lost alongside the loss of the child's life. *Better Care, Better Lives* (Department of Health 2008c) outlines a strategy for future children's palliative care services that argues strongly for increased choice for children and families in relation to place of care. The realization of this requires not only an expansion of community services but considerable flexibility on the part of hospital services to outreach their medical and nursing expertise, by joint home and community visits and the provision of telephone and other modes of clinical advice accessible to community teams and families on a 24-hour basis.

Conclusion

In supporting families caring for technology-dependent children at home, knowledge of services available and funding mechanisms need to interface with appropriate assessments of individual need to ensure flexible packages of care are developed. There is a considerable body of evidence on the experiences of parents caring for technology-dependent children outside of the hospital setting and the tensions present within current services. In addition an increasingly robust policy literature is available to guide practitioners and commissioners on appropriate service provision. There is a further need to investigate the experiences of children themselves, in home, school and respite settings to develop the knowledge base of practitioners in this expanding field of child health practice.

Finally researchers, educators and workforce planners need to address the experiences and needs of the professionals providing care for this group of children (Hewitt-Taylor 2008). This information is required in order to develop an appropriate children's workforce that is skilled, sustainable and delivers care that responds to the non-static needs of children and families. The policy agenda makes it clear that well-coordinated, mult-iagency work is a necessary requirement to fulfil the *Every Child Matters* agenda; however, as yet relatively little attention is paid to training and recruiting a workforce equipped for this task. The examples provided in this chapter raise questions about how community staff can develop and maintain skills in high dependency care when they are exposed to only a small cohort of children, and how can high dependency care staff respond to children and families for whom care at home may be provided by lay carers and expert parents when they are admitted to hospital for acute care episodes. The Department for Children, Families and Schools (2009) published its strategy for developing an appropriate children's workforce by 2020. They advocate a combined strategic and local approach to ensuring that developments reflect local needs and can access the specialist knowledge and resources located strategically. High dependency staff in the hospital and community need to ensure that they are able to influence this process.

As the plans for developing health care outlined in Lord Darzi's next stage review (Department of Health 2008d) begin to change service provision towards further centralization in children's inpatient services, with the majority of local services being community and ambulatory, the challenges of managing local-based care for technology-dependent children may require alternative models of linking services based in more geographically distant inpatient high dependency units. The strategy for children's health, *Healthy Lives, Brighter Futures* (Department of Health 2009) confirms the expectation that community children's nursing services are the foundation for local service provision for children with long-term conditions and complex health needs. As this chapter has illustrated, children who have high dependency needs therefore require strong links to the hospital services, with a cohort of technology-dependent children forming a significant part of the workload for these services.

 Learning activities

- Review the principles of respiratory assessment and consider the implications of conducting this in the home setting. What guidance would you give to non-nurse carers of a child with a tracheostomy on the recognition of changes in respiratory function?
- Recall Sayed's father's comments on the education he received and consider how you might prepare and support parents for the emotional and social impact of caring for a technology-dependent child.
- Consider the multidisciplinary resources required to provide services to enable a technology-dependent child from your own practice meet the *Every Child Matters* outcomes. How could you present the service costs of these resources to a commissioning authority?
- Reflect on your own practice in relation to negotiating care activities with families of children dependent on technology: who decides on 'parenting' and 'nursing' roles and boundaries? Review Kirk *et al.* (2005) and Alderson (2006) in the light of your own practice.

References and further reading

ACT (2007) *The Transition Care Pathway: a framework for the development of integrated multiagency care pathways for young people with life-threatening and life-limiting conditions.* ACT – The Association for Children's Palliative Care, Bristol.

Alderson P (2006) Parents' consent to neonatal decisions about feeding and discharge. *Journal of Neonatal Nursing* **12**: 6–13.

Beresford B, Clarke S, Sloper P (2005) *Integrating Services for Disabled Children, Young People and their Families in York: Consultation Project.* Social Policy Research Unit, University of York.

Bush A, Fraser J, Jardine E, Paton J, Simmonds A, Wallis C (2005) Respiratory management of the infant with type 1 spinal muscular atrophy. *Archives of Disease in Childhood* **90**: 709–711.

Carnevale FA, Alexander E, Davis M, Rennick JE, Troini R (2006) Daily living with distress and enrichment: the moral experiences of families with ventilator assisted children at home. *Pediatrics* **117**(1): 48–60.

Carnevale FA, Rehm RS, Kirk S, McKeever S (2008) What we know (and do not know) about raising children with complex and continuing care needs. *Journal of Child Health Care* **12**(4): 4–6.

Cejer B (2007) The needs and experiences of long-term ventilator children and their families. *Paediatric Nursing* **19**(5): 42–45.

Department for Education and Skills/Department of Health (2006a) *Framework for the Joint Planning of Children's and Young People's Services.* DfES and DH. HMSO.

Department for Education and Skills/Department of Health (2006b) *Transition: getting it right for young people.* HMSO.

Department of Health (2000) *Framework for the Assessment of Children in Need and Their Families.* The Stationery Office, London.

Department of Health (2004a) *National Service Framework for Children, Young People and Maternity Services: children and young people who are ill.* www.doh.gov.uk/nsf/children.htm (accessed 12 August 2007).

Department of Health (2004b) *National Service Framework for Children, Young People and Maternity Services: acquired brain injury exemplar.* Department of Health. HMSO.

Department of Health (2005a) *Complex disability exemplar. National Service Framework for Children, Young People and Maternity Services.* Department of Health. HMSO.

Department of Health (2005b) *Long term ventilation exemplar. National Service Framework for Children, Young People and Maternity Services.* Department of Health. HMSO.

Department of Health (2008a) *A National Framework for Assessing Children's Continuing Care.* Partnership for Children, Families and Maternity. HMSO.

Department of Health (2008b) *Aiming High for Disabled Children: short breaks implementation guidance.* Available at www.everychildmatters.gov.uk/ahdc (accessed 11 November 2008).

Department of Health (2008c) *Better Care, Better Lives.* HMSO.

Department of Health (2008d) *High Quality Care for All: NHS the next stage review final report.* HMSO.

Department of Health/Department for Children, Schools and Families (2009) *Healthy Lives, Brighter Futures: the strategy for children and young people's health.* HMSO.

Eaton N (2001) Models of community children's nursing. *Paediatric Nursing* **13**(1): 32–36.

Elston S (2003) *Assessment of Children with Life-Limiting Conditions and Their Families: a guide to effective care planning.* ACT, Bristol.

Gillis J (2008) 'We want everything done.' *Archives of Disease in Childhood* **93**: 192–193.

Glendinning C, Kirk S, Guiffrida A, Lawton D (2001) Technology dependent children in the community: definitions, numbers and costs. *Child: Care, Health & Development* **27**(4): 321–324.

Graham RJ, Pemstein DM, Palfrey JS (2008) Included but isolated: early intervention programmes provision for children and families with chronic respiratory support needs. *Child: Care, Health & Development* **34**(3): 373–379.

Green S (2007) 'We're tired not sad': benefits and burdens of mothering a child with a disability. *Social Science and Medicine* **64**: 150–163.

Harrison G, Beresford M, Shaw NJ (2006) Acute life threatening events among infants on home oxygen. *Paediatric Nursing* **18**(1): 27–29.

Heaton J, Noyes J, Sloper P, Shah R (2005) Families experiences of caring for technology dependent children: a temporal perspective. *Health and Social Care in the Community* **13**(5): 441–450.

Heaton J, Noyes J, Sloper P, Shah R (2006) The experience of sleep disruption in families of technology dependent children living at home. *Children and Society* **20**: 196–208.

Hewitt-Taylor J (2008) Working in the family home. Chapter 5 in *Providing Support at Home for Children and Young People who have Complex Health Needs.* Wiley, London: 70–82.

Holden C (2001) Review of home paediatric parenteral nutrition in the UK. *British Journal of Nursing* **10**(12): 782–788.

Horrocks S, Somerset M, Salisbury C (2002) Do children with non-malignant life-threatening conditions receive effective palliative care? A pragmatic evaluation of a local service. *Palliative Medicine* **16**: 410–416.

Jardine E, Wallis C (1998) Core guidelines for the discharge home of long-term assisted ventilation patients in the United Kingdom. *Thorax* **53**: 762–767.

Kakazanov V, Monagle P, Chan K (2008) Thromboembolisim in infants and children with gastrointestinal failure receiving long-term parenteral nutrition. *Journal of Parenteral and Enteral Nutrition* **32**(1): 88–93.

Kirk S, Glendinning C (2004) Developing services to support parents caring for a technology-dependant child at home. *Child: Care, Health and Development* **30**(3): 209–218.

Kirk S, Glendinning C, Callery P (2005) Parent or nurse? The experience of being a parent of a technology-dependent child. *Journal of Advanced Nursing* **51**(5): 456–464.

Koglmeier J, Day C, Puntis J (2008) Clinical outcome in patients from a single region dependent on parenteral nutrition for 28 days or more. *Archives of Disease in Childhood* **93**: 300–302.

Lenton S, Frank L, Salt A (2004) Children with complex health care needs supporting the child and family in the community. *Child: Care, Health and Development* **30**(3): 191–192.

Liben S, Papadatou D, Wolfe J (2008) Paediatric palliative care: challenges and emerging ideas. *Lancet* **371**: 852–864.

MacDonald H, Callery P (2004) Different meanings of respite: a study of parents, nurses and social workers caring for children with complex needs. *Child: Care, Health and Development* **30**(3): 279–288.

Margolan H, Fraser J, Lenton S (2004) Parental experience of services when their child requires long-term ventilation: implications for commissioning and providing services. *Child: Care, Health and Development* **30**(3): 257–264.

Muir J, Dryden S (2000) Collaborative planning for children with chronic, complex care needs. In Muir J, Sidey A (eds) *A Textbook of Community Children's Nursing*. Bailliere Tindall, Edinburgh and New York: 216–222.

Murphy G (2001) The technology dependant child at home (Parts 1&2). *Paediatric Nursing* **13**(7&8).

Noyes J (2002) Barriers that delay children and young people who are dependent on mechanical ventilation from being discharged from hospital. *Journal of Clinical Nursing* **11**(1): 2–11.

Noyes J, Lewis M (2005) *From Hospital to Home: guidance on the discharge management and community support for children using long-term ventilation.* Barnado's, Barkingside, Essex.

Noyes J, Lewis M (2007) Compiling, costing and funding complex packages of home-based healthcare. *Paediatric Nursing* **19**(9): 28–32.

Noyes J, Godfrey C, Beecham J (2006) Resource use and service costs for ventilator dependant children and young people in the UK. *Health and Social Care in the Community* **14**(6): 508–522.

Parker D, Maddocks I, Stern LM (1999) The role of palliative care in advanced muscular dystrophy and spinal muscular atrophy. *Journal of Paediatric and Child Health* **35**(3): 245–250.

Royal College of Nursing (2008) *Managing Children with Health Care Needs: delegation of clinical procedures training and accountability issues.* http//.www.rcn. org.uk (accessed 22 February 2008).

Ryder M (2006) Evidenced based practice in the management of vascular access devices for home parenteral nutrition therapy. *Journal of Parenteral and Enteral Nutrition* **30**(1): 82–93.

Stanley K (2008) *Having a Break: good practice in short breaks for families with children who have complex needs and disability.* Social Care Institute for Excellence.

Stephens N (2005) Complex care packages: supporting seamless discharge for the child and family. *Paediatric Nursing* **16**(7): 30–32.

Thornley E (2008) Commissioning care of children with complex needs. In Teare J (ed.) *Caring for Children with Complex Needs in the Community.* Blackwell Publishing, Oxford: 21–34.

Thurgate C (2005) Respite for children with complex health needs. *Paediatric Nursing* **17**(3): 14–18.

Wagner J, Power EJ, Fox H (1988) *Technology dependent children: hospital versus home care.* Office of Technology Assessment Task Force. JP Lippincott, Philadelphia.

While A, Cockett A, Lewis S (2004) Children and young people requiring home assisted ventilation in the south of England: incidence, receipt of care support and components of the care package. *Children and Society* **18**: 207–217.

Willis E (2007) Symptom care flowcharts: a case study *Paediatric Nursing* **19**(1): 14–17.

Wray D (2008) Educational support for children with complex care needs. In Teare J (ed.) *Caring for Children with Complex Needs in the Community.* Blackwell Publishing, Oxford: 167–187.

Yantzi NM, Rosenberg MW, McKeever P (2006) Getting out of the house: the challenges mothers face when their children have long-term care needs. *Health and Social Care in the Community* **15**(1): 45–55.

11

Mental health and intellectual impairment

Louise Clark

Learning outcomes

- To develop an understanding of the concept of mental health and intellectual impairment and how this may have a bearing on nursing care
- To study the basic framework of mental health assessment
- To develop an understanding of caring for these patient groups in the acute environment

Introduction

Children and adolescents with mental health problems form a sizable portion of patients in a high dependency situation, as indeed do those who have intellectual impairments (sometimes otherwise known as global developmental delays or special needs). This chapter will examine a variety of conditions observed in some of these children and adolescents and will demonstrate the importance for children's nurses to develop a broad overview of some of the appropriate systems of care and management. The standard mental health assessment process, otherwise known as 'formulation', which is undertaken by specially trained paediatric mental health professionals will be discussed. However this should not be considered as a full and explicit guidance of how to perform the assessment, simply an overview for the non-mental-health professional. Developmental issues which affect both the diagnosis and management of children with mental health problems and/or intellectual impairment will be explored, as will be some of the most common situations where mental health or intellectual impairment result in the high dependency situation.

The formulation process

This is the standard mental health assessment which is utilized for all patients and is carried out by specially trained mental health professionals. Certain adaptations are made to the process dependent on the age of the child and their developmental level. As with other forms of assessment, consent is required from the child or adolescent's parents or guardians if they are too young to provide their own permission.

The process consists of four distinct parts:

1. History taking
2. Full physical assessment
3. Mental state examination
4. Formulation.

History

Collateral information from parents or carers is important, especially when the child is very young and cannot articulate their thoughts and feelings easily. A picture of pre-morbid functioning is essential to the diagnostic process. A complete developmental, educational, medical and psychiatric history is essential, as is an indirect assessment of the parents' personalities, their relationship with each other and their parenting styles. Family social, medical and psychiatric history provides an intrinsic part of this stage in the assessment process.

Child protection issues (including the identification of children at risk of emotional abuse) should always be at the forefront of the clinician's mind in such interviews.

Abused children often present with the symptoms of depression, suicidal behaviour and/or post-traumatic stress disorder if they are victims.

An interview with the child or adolescent with or without the parents then follows.

Learning disabilities, pervasive developmental disorders (e.g. autism, Rett syndrome) and adult disorders with roots in adolescence must be identified as such conditions may both skew and/or complicate any diagnosis. Some medical conditions may also have an impact on mental health diagnosis such as diabetes, degenerative conditions, epilepsy and other neurological conditions. Current medication must be identified as this may also have an impact on the child's presenting complaint.

Physical assessment

This process is a vital component of any mental health assessment and should constitute a review of all systems: cardiovascular, gastrointestinal, genito-urinary, respiratory, neurological, sensory and musculoskeletal. In addition height, weight and waist measurements should be performed. Where indicated, specialist scans may be needed such as x-rays, bone scans, magnetic resonance imaging (MRI), electroencephalography (EEG) or electrocardiogram (ECG).

With adolescents the impact of lifestyle factors must be taken in to account such as alcohol and illicit substance abuse, diet, sexual health and exercise routine. Adolescents are not always totally forthcoming with some of this information, but consent for a urine test in the case of suspected illicit drug use may be indicated. Blood screening for full haematology and urea and electrolytes (U&Es) is always recommended, with hormonal screening performed if needed (glucose, pancreatic function, thyroid function and T4, steroid and sex hormones, etc.). The use of a malnutrition assessment tool may also be indicated.

Mental state examination

The mental state examination (MSE) provides a 'snap-shot' of an individual at the time of the interview and is subject to the interpretation of the assessor. It is based on distinct areas which may hold diagnostic clues and much of this assessment is achieved through subtle observation and questioning by the assessor.

Appearance

- Correct developmental stage for age?
- Overweight or underweight?
- Are they and their clothes clean?
- Evidence of injury such as self harm or physical abuse by others (e.g. scaring on arms, burn marks)?
- Evidence of dysmorphic features?
- Do they smell of body odour, alcohol or smoke?

Behaviour

- Does their motor behaviour appear normal, is there any suggestion of a tremor, tic or twitch?
- Do they seem suspicious, fearful, or display catatonic features?
- Are they sitting or lying still, or do they seem agitated or fidgety?

Rapport

- Does the child make eye contact?
- Do they seem comfortable to chat?
- Are they co-operative, defensive, aggressive, fearful or confused?
- Do they smile or cry?
- Is their attitude inappropriate to the context of the interview?

Speech

- What is the volume and the speed of their speech like?
- Does the speech have an unusual rhythm?
- Do they have a stutter?
- Do they speak incoherently and make little or no sense?

Mood and affect

- Do they appear depressed, anxious, elated, frightened or angry?
- Is the appropriateness of the observed mood applicable to the reported mood?
- Is the affect within a normal range to the mood reported? Affect may be observed by measuring the person's posture, expression, speech and reactivity.

Perception

- Are abnormal perceptions genuine hallucinations or delusions, or intrusive thoughts?
- Which sensory organ do the hallucinations come from?
- If there are auditory hallucinations present, are they elementary or complex?
- Are auditory hallucinations, if complex, experienced in the first, second or third person?
- Do they seem to be experiencing or responding to hallucinations during the interview?

Thinking

- Do there seem to be abnormal beliefs and disorganized thinking?
- Do delusions appear to be primary or secondary?

- What is the content of the delusion?
- Is the delusion mood congruent?
- Does echolalia, idiosyncratic word use, irrelevant answers, thought blocking, or flight of ideas seem apparent?

> **Remember**
> A delusion is a falsely held belief, held on illogical grounds, therefore someone cannot complain of having a delusion or a hallucination, it is up to others to observe them.

Cognition

- Does the child or adolescent appear to be drowsy, alert or hyper-vigilant?
- Do they appear to have an intellectual impairment?
- Are they intoxicated through alcohol or drugs?
- Is cognition affected in other ways?

Cognitive tests are generally indicated in children and adolescents in order to establish the cognitive developmental level, memory, recall and degree of consciousness.

Insight

- Does the patient think they have a mental health problem?
- Are they in denial of any mental health issues?
- Do they realize the seriousness of their condition?
- Do they think they need treatment?
- Will they accept treatment?

Suicidal ideation

- Do they feel that they no longer want to live?
- Have they thought of taking their own life?
- If so, have they planned how this will be done?
- How far have they got with the planning process?

Obviously these are not questions that the clinician will ask the child or adolescent in an outright manner. Caution, skill, observation and practice are essential components in the successful procurement of this information.

Formulation: presentation of the case

'Formulation' is a term used in mental health services by psychiatrists to give a summary and understand the patient's problems.

Having studied all the other areas of the assessment process, a picture emerges and it is sensible to categorize findings in six distinct areas.

Description

Here identifying information is listed along with the main features of the presenting complaint and previous medical, psychiatric and family history. Any abnormalities from the physical assessment and positive findings from the mental state examination are noted.

Differential and preferred diagnosis

Differential diagnoses are listed in order of probability. Only conditions that are supported by clinical evidence during assessment should be noted, with reasons given for each alternative choice.

Aetiology

The aetiology of many mental health disorders is often problematic to define. Very often a bio-psychological perspective must be adopted in order to pinpoint what predisposed to the condition. It is important to attempt to identify not only the predisposing factors but also those that precipitated it and those that will perpetuate the problem if unaddressed.

Management

A management plan adopting a bio-psychosocial approach should be established at this point utilizing a child-centred focus. This should cover both short- and long-term needs and also cover any further investigations or specialist input required. Due to the complexities of multi-aetiology in many children who have mental health problems, management requires specialist input from Child and Adolescent Mental Health Services (CAMHS) in a great number of cases. Priorities around nursing care should always focus on safeguarding the child and managing the immediate physical problems.

Prognosis

The natural expected course of the condition is established here in addition to factors which may complicate the process.

Risk assessment

This process is of vital importance when the child or adolescent is suspected of having either a mental health problem or intellectual impairment and where there could be the added risk of challenging behaviour, aggression or violence. Safety issues must be considered especially in relation to the child, other patients, staff and visitors. In some clinical areas standard tools exist; however, often such assessments need to be tailor made. The risk assessment is predominantly the responsibility of nursing staff and should broadly consist of thee distinct areas:

What is the risk?
This can be determined by speaking to parents and carers and by observation. It may be the risk of aggression, violence or self harm which can increase when the child or adolescent is frightened or stressed.

How can the risk be reduced, if not eliminated?
It is helpful to identify what methods are used in the home environment and then adapt them to the ward or unit. If the child is prone to challenging or dangerous behaviour, nursing them away from others is an option unless of course the child is at risk of self harm or a suicide attempt. In extreme cases one-to-one nursing may be indicated. Behavioural charts may be a useful management tool in such cases such as ABC charts:

A   Antecedent: What happened immediately before the challenging behaviour happened, where did it happen and who was present? – otherwise known as the 'trigger'. Obviously this is recorded retrospectively.
B   Behaviour: What did the behaviour consist of?
C   Consequence: How was the situation handled and by whom?

The importance of such charts is to build up an accurate picture of the trigger factors and to subsequently deduce the best possible way of preventing and managing untoward events. However, teams must be diligent in recording all events in detail in order for such charts to be effective.

What is the emergency procedure?
This section broadly outlines measures that will be employed in the event of a 'worst case scenario'. This may cause management issues on paediatric units if violence needs to be contained, as nurses must balance their duty of care against often being untrained in the holding (or restraint) of patients. The use of such measures when employed by staff who have not received specific training in this area may be construed as assault (Lyon and Pimor 2004). Often, therefore, when situations escalate beyond control there is no option other than to call for security staff.

Child abuse

Many factors have been recognized as indicators for child abuse which can result in emotional and/or physical neglect of the child or in actual physical injury or sexual abuse.

In addition to the physical manifestations of abuse, children may present with the signs and symptoms of depression, anxiety, failure to thrive, aggression and other challenging behaviours, suicidal behaviour, post-traumatic stress disorder or precocious sexual behaviour.

This is a difficult diagnosis to make but if there are suspicions of child abuse the nurse must remember that the child's safety is the main priority and there should be a low threshold for informing social services if suspicions are raised.

For a more indepth discussion of the mental health assessment and formulation process the reader is directed to *The Shorter Oxford Textbook of Psychiatry* (Gelder *et al.* 2001).

Developmental issues

'Normal' development in children and adolescents varies a great deal. However, in children who have intellectual impairments development may be dramatically delayed, and in some areas may never occur. When utilizing a bio-psychosocial approach with some of these children and adolescents it becomes evident that there are marked differences between them in areas that have been affected. For example, especially in children with autism, there may be areas of near brilliance, such as with music or mathematics, but their emotional development may show serious immaturity. Other children with autism may be totally developmentally delayed in all areas.

Children who have intellectual impairment are more prone to epilepsy, autism and psychosis, the latter not usually developing until late adolescence. It is considered that such conditions are more prevalent in these children due to damage of the brain. Diagnostic overshadowing may occur in that other conditions are ignored or remain uninvestigated as the symptoms are ascribed to the intellectual impairment or considered to be 'behavioural' in origin.

Some autistic spectrum disorders, including Asperger syndrome, are not always diagnosed in childhood and are difficult to diagnose during adolescence due to considerable problems surrounding co-morbidity (Gillberg 2003). It is not uncommon for teenagers with autistic spectrum disorders to experience mild to moderate depression and irritability and to indulge in antisocial activities. For a diagnosis of autism there should be no clinically significant developmental delay in spoken or receptive language, cognition or self-help skills; adaptive behaviour and curiosity about the environment should be consistent with normal intellectual development during the first three years of life (World Health Organization 1992).

Some children who have intellectual impairment may display excellent social skills, this can mask the true extent of their disability as other areas of cognition can then be assumed to be functioning at a higher level than they actually are.

The term 'adaptive functioning' is useful when attempting to establish a child's ability and developmental stage. Intelligence quotient (IQ) alone is inconclusive and does not take into account other abilities or disabilities that may not seem immediately evident but which could have a great impact on overall performance. For example, a child may have an IQ of 85 (above the considered level for intellectual impairment to be considered present) but may have sensory or motor problems which could be a barrier to learning and result in them functioning as if they had an IQ well below 85. Mental health problems in children with or without intellectual impairment will generally have an impact on their adaptive functioning. Other factors may also influence IQ testing such as stress, tiredness and a short concentration span (Burke and Cigno 2000).

The hyperkinetic disorders (e.g. attention deficit disorder and attention deficit hyperactivity disorder) have an early onset, usually in the first five years of life, and may affect children at all intellectual levels. This group of conditions are characterized by inattention, impulsivity and recklessness with excessive activity. These children often find themselves in disciplinary trouble because of breaches of rules due to lack of thought rather than deliberate defiance. In comparison, oppositional defiant disorder is characterized by tantrums, swearing and stubbornness and is easily recognizable. Conduct disorder is a more pervasive condition which is antisocial in tendency and is characterized by aggression, destruction of property, deceitfulness and serious violation of rules. It has been observed that many children diagnosed with oppositional defiant disorder or conduct disorder proceed to cluster B personality disorders in adulthood, so it is important that a diagnosis is made and therapeutic interventions are put in place.

Distinguishing between behavioural disturbance and psychiatric disorders in children and adolescents is problematic, especially if there is also intellectual impairment present; empirical and conceptual issues relating to the nature of disorders questions both the reliability and validity of a psychiatric diagnosis. Other issues such as high rates of acquiescence in certain interview situations with children and adolescents may also skew the diagnostic process (Kroese *et al.* 2000).

Case study 1: 14-year-old with developmental delay

Sophie Miller is a 14-year-old girl who has been admitted to your ward for investigations and management of epilepsy. She has a mild to moderate global developmental delay and the possibility of a diagnosis of psychosis has also been mooted due to an increase in bizarre behaviours and the sudden onset of conversations with an imaginary friend.

Sophie does have some violent outbursts both at home and in the mainstream school that she attends with support. These incidents include kicking, biting and damage to property. She has a strong dislike of unknown males and has been known to spit at them for no apparent reason, often in public places. She has absconded from both home and school on many occasions, usually when she is frightened for one reason or another.

Whilst in hospital she will be accompanied by her mother whenever possible who works full time and will continue to do so throughout Sophie's stay, so will realistically only be there in the evenings and at the weekends. Sophie's mother is a single parent and there are no siblings.

Management

1. With the limited information available, compile a risk assessment and management plan.
2. Who should be involved in Sophie's care throughout her stay on the ward and where can you get help, advice and guidance to ensure that she is properly cared for?
3. Look at the seizure charts that are available in your ward or department. Are they accurately completed by staff? Is there sufficient information recorded on them for clinicians to establish an accurate pattern of seizure activity?

It is important to remember that some types of seizures may be confused with the bizarre behaviours which are sometimes seen in people who have severe intellectual impairments. Conditions such as schizophrenia and other psychoses (which are believed to be more prevalent in this group of adolescents) are also problematic to diagnose as they are unable to undergo the full formulation process due to communication issues and lack of co-operation. This situation is often compounded by the frequent presence of epilepsy, which occurs more commonly in people who have damage to the brain; the more severe the intellectual impairment the more likely the person is to have epilepsy.

Some common mental health conditions

The huge variety of mental health and intellectual impairment conditions mean that the area can only be touched upon in this short chapter. Some of the more common conditions such as attempted suicide, self harm and substance abuse, as well as caring for the child or adolescent who is suspected to be suffering from first-onset psychosis, are seen with regularity on acute wards and units. The importance of close working with the CAMHS cannot be over-emphasized. Assessment, care planning, implementation and monitoring should all be viewed utilizing a bio-psychosocial approach between the multidisciplinary teams. Sometimes children and adolescents are admitted who are already known to community psychiatric or learning disability services and their involvement is strongly recommended. It is part of the changing role of the community learning mental health and disability teams to give advice and guidance to generic NHS services (Department of Health 2001), and this also applies when the child is admitted to hospital.

Case study 2: 14-year-old who has self harmed

Jamie is a 14-year-old boy who lives with his divorced mother and two younger twin sisters (aged 12) in a high-rise block of inner city flats. He is admitted to your ward following a suicide attempt where he took copious amounts of alcohol, paracetamol and diazepam together with his ongoing consumption of cannabis. He left a suicide note stating that life was hopeless and he could not continue with it.

Jamie has had a problematic childhood, he has often played truant from school and has been in trouble with the police for shoplifting, alcohol and illicit substance abuse, and for carrying a knife.

Management

1. What are the immediate issues associated with Jamie's suicide attempt?
2. What do you think may have predisposed and precipitated the attempt?
3. Provide a comprehensive risk assessment which will cover his time in hospital.
4. To whom should Jamie and/or his family be referred on discharge and what are the risk factors on discharge? Give suggestions as to how these factors may be reduced and managed.
5. What issues may perpetuate Jamie's problems if they remain unresolved?

Substance abuse

The scenario presented is sadly not an unusual one. It is known that adolescents who habitually use illegal substances have a tendency to participate in other high-risk activities (Lavery *et al.* 1993) and there is evidence that this could stem from a host of risk factors either inherent in the personality, interpersonal relationships or the surrounding environment (Steinberg 1996). Many of these young people carry some of these behaviours in to adulthood (Kelly 2000). Several factors have been identified as contributory towards attempted suicide in adolescence including impulsivity (Kingsbury *et al.* 1999), issues with problem solving (Hawton *et al.* 1999), hopelessness (Kerfoot 1996), hostility and anger (Simmonds *et al.* 1991). Psychiatric disorders carry an increased risk of suicidal behaviour in adolescents with depression being one of the most common causes (Burgess *et al.* 1998). Management of care and treatment for children and adolescents should always follow NICE (National Institute for Clinical Excellence) guidelines relevant to that particular condition. These guidelines for the management of care differ to those set out for adults who have similar conditions. Where medication is necessary, for instance in the case of depression or psychosis, patients and their parents or carers should be informed of the rationale for drug treatment, the time course of the treatment, possible side effects, the need to take the medication as prescribed and the delay in onset of effect of the medication.

Academic failure and a disconnection with school are associated with adolescent drug use (Ary *et al.* 1999) and attendance at school and attempting to increase performance are at the heart of family-based therapy between adolescents and parents. The CAMHS may also be utilized in providing support to the adolescent, and engagement with them while still in hospital is recommended.

Emotional disorders

Emotional disorders are marked by anxiety or depression and are sometimes observed as developmental delays rather than an illness in themselves. The prognosis is often good if a diagnosis is made and treatment is given. Phobic anxiety disorder, social anxiety disorder and separation anxiety disorder are all common conditions within this group and can cause distress for both the child concerned and, indeed, to the family as a whole.

Eating disorders

Eating disorders are far more common in females than in males and their prevalence is rising. Anorexia nervosa has an earlier onset than that of bulimia nervosa and there is a high incidence of other conditions which accompany them, for example mood disorders, substance abuse and self harm. Children with anorexia nervosa may become critically ill and require admission in some cases, where preferable to a specialist unit, but sometimes they may be admitted to general paediatric wards. Hospitalization is usually considered necessary when the body mass index is less than $13.5\,kg/m^2$, there is sudden dramatic weight loss, severe electrolyte imbalance or associated mental health problems such as suicidal risk factors. The condition may also be observed when children are admitted with unrelated complaints.

Several factors have been ascribed as contributory to both anorexia nervosa and bulimia nervosa, including Western society's obsession with being thin and the media contribution toward this, genetic issues, overprotection, the push to succeed by professional class parents and attempts by pubescent girls to avoid their changing body shape and menstruation.

Anorexia nervosa is characterized by deliberate weight loss which is induced and sustained by the patient and has its first onset most commonly in adolescence or young adulthood. A persistent dread of being fat persists as an intrusive overvalued idea (World Health Organization 1992) which results in a self-imposed low weight threshold. In order for a diagnosis to be made the individual must display a weight loss, or a lack of weight gain which is self induced, the body weight must be at least 15% below the normal or expected weight for the child's age and height, females with this condition usually cease menstruation. Other features may also be present including self-induced vomiting, purging, excessive exercise, and the use of appetite suppressants and/or diuretics. If the onset is prepubertal, puberty may be delayed or arrested, but with recovery puberty is often completed normally, but menarche is late. The management of anorexia nervosa is problematic due to the patient's ambivalence towards treatment and must therefore follow a collaborative and therapeutic alliance from the first point of contact with services; motivational interviewing has been shown to be helpful.

Bulimia nervosa is characterized by recurrent episodes of overeating large amounts of food in short periods of time (at least twice a week over a period of three months, in order to qualify for a diagnosis; World Health Organization 1992). There is a persistent preoccupation with food and a strong compulsion to eat, however the individual will counteract the excess calories by either self-induced vomiting or purging, alternating with periods of starvation, excessive exercise or the use of drugs which are obtained illegally, including diuretics, appetite suppressants or thyroxine-based drugs. People who have bulimia are usually of a healthy weight. Treatment given is psychologically based with specialist eating disorder input or inpatient care given in severe cases. Antidepressant therapy, particularly the tricyclic antidepressants and SSRIs (selective serotonin reuptake inhibitors) have been shown to be useful in the reduction of binge eating and purging behaviour.

Other eating disorders which fulfil some of the features of anorexia or bulimia nervosa but not enough to warrant a diagnosis may be seen, and are usually known as atypical or unspecified eating disorders.

Mood disorders

Although more serious conditions such as bipolar disorder may develop in adolescence, by far the most common mood disorder observed at this time of life is depression. This condition can largely be divided in to two distinct types, that which is sometimes known as a biological depression (otherwise referred to as endogenous or somatic) in its nature, and that which is reactive in its context (also known as adjustment disorder). Biological depression is diagnosable when there are no known environmental reasons for the depression and there is a visible clinical picture. Reactive depression is diagnosable when there are understandable reasons for the person to be depressed due to adverse psychological circumstances.

Whatever the cause of the depressed mood (biological or reactive), depression is classified as being mild, moderate or severe and the diagnosis of category depends on the individual's fulfilment of a list of symptoms, their duration and severity; these include a loss of interest in normally pleasurable activities, decreased energy, a change in sleep and eating patterns, weight loss or gain, loss of confidence, feelings of guilt and self reproach and inability to concentrate (World Health Organization 1992). Children and young people who have suffered recent bereavement or parental separation are potentially at risk of depression, as are those who are victims of bullying, abuse or abnormal psychological situations. Children and young people who use alcohol or certain substances are also more prone to depression, often due to the chemical compounds present.

Children and young people who are suspected of suffering from depression should always undergo the full mental health assessment (formulation) including a full physical assessment in order to make a conclusive diagnosis. Particular attention should be paid to thyroid function levels as the symptoms of an underactive thyroid may mirror those of a depressive illness.

The management and treatment of depression are governed by National Institute of Clinical Excellence (NICE) guidelines and are specific to children and adolescents.

Destructive behaviour

For many adolescents there is an element of destructive health behaviour which includes drinking alcohol, smoking and illicit substance abuse. Cannabis and ecstasy are commonly used and about 5% of teenagers are estimated to experiment with more serious drugs including cocaine, heroin, amphetamines and solvents. Signs of illicit substance abuse may include mood changes, loss of appetite, failure to achieve their normal academic standards, loss of interest in leisure pursuits, drowsiness, furtive behaviour and delinquent behaviour which may result in prosecution. Irresponsible sexual behaviour is also common at this stage of life with many not using contraception initially. Health promotion in schools, supportive families and access to the relevant health professionals is essential at this time of high-risk behaviour. When discussing sensitive issues with adolescents it is important to:

- take the time to listen
- respect their need for privacy
- avoid judgemental attitudes
- assure confidentiality (but explain that in extreme circumstances this may have to be broken)

enable them to arrive at the solution to the problem themselves, don't lecture!

Suicide or self harm

Young people who are depressed sometimes have thoughts of death or harming themselves; often the initial point of contact with health services may be through self harm or a suicide attempt (parasuicide).

The term 'self harm' relates to a myriad of actions including self poisoning (overdosing with the intent to kill oneself), self injury (cutting, burning, excessive scratching or skin picking, etc.) or, in the extreme, attempted or actual suicide.

In attempting to establish the seriousness of the suicide attempt the 'formulation' process is at the heart of the assessment process, although it is not always possible to perform this on admission to hospital as it is dependent on the seriousness of the patient's clinical condition.

Four key points are intrinsic to establishing the seriousness of the attempt and the subsequent risk assessment process:

1. Was the attempt planned in advance? Fatal suicide attempts often take weeks or months of intricate planning, suicide notes or letters are sometimes written, other less serious attempts may be preceded by the consumption of drugs or alcohol.
2. Were precautions taken to avoid discovery?
3. Was a dangerous method adopted? It has been known for some time that males will use more violent methods than females, for example: jumping under trains, hanging or shooting. This suicidal behaviour difference is often apparent in adolescence; however, it must be noted that in terms of self-poisoning many children and adolescents are unaware of the amount of drugs or medication that would be necessary to procure a successful suicide attempt.
4. Was help sought immediately after the attempt? Some people will seek help soon after the event when they realize the gravity of their actions.

For children and adolescents who harm themselves help and advice must be sought from the CAMHS team as soon as possible; children's nurses can then work alongside the team in order to secure the best possible patient outcome.

First-onset psychosis

Schizophrenia is arguably the most common form of psychosis. It is rarely seen in childhood but may have its first onset in adolescence (more frequently at this age in males rather than females). There is a genetic link and it does run in families; brain abnormalities, both structural and functional, can be found in individuals who suffer from schizophrenia. Stressful life events have been shown to precipitate the first onset of the illness, hence adolescence is a time when this can happen.

Schizophrenia is characterized by a number of features including:

- *Delusions:* these are unshakable false beliefs which are held with certainty. Despite evidence to the contrary the person will not recognize reality (culture and religion must be taken into account before identification of delusions is made).
- *Hallucinations:* a perception that arises despite a stimulus being present via one of the sensory organs (the most common are auditory or visual hallucinations).

The initial treatment depends on the setting and the severity of the illness; where possible adolescents are treated in the community. However, there is a significant risk that the symptoms of first-onset psychosis may lead to self harm or self neglect and hospitalization is sometimes needed, ideally this should be on a CAMHS unit where specialist care can be given. This is not always an option and occasionally patients are admitted to adult mental health units or to paediatric wards (in the case of younger adolescents especially); when the latter occurs, support should be sought immediately from CAMHS services.

Other forms of psychosis must be excluded before a diagnosis of schizophrenia can be made. These include:

- drug-induced psychosis (as occurs sometimes with cannabis and becoming more common in first-onset adolescent psychotic episodes seen by CAMHS)
- bipolar disorder
- delusional disorders
- schizotypal disorder
- schizoaffective disorder
- organic behaviour disorder (as seen in young people who have severe intellectual impairments).

Due to the intricacies of the diagnostic process the initial 'blanket' term that is generally applied is that of first-onset psychosis. It can usually take a long period of time before the exact subgroup of the condition is arrived at. It is of vital importance that, where possible, young people are not 'labelled' as suffering from a mental health problem in order to avoid stigma, but this does have to be balanced against the need for them to receive the necessary services at the earliest possible juncture.

Support is essential for the whole family in the case of first-onset psychosis in terms of education, management and treatment, and of connecting them to networks and systems that are available to the family as a whole.

Conclusion

There is certainly an increase in child and adolescent mental health problems in recent years and often they will present with a complex myriad of issues. The care of these young people whilst in acute paediatric services requires delicate handling and should always involve CAMHS who can provide advice and suggestions to the child health team. Thorough mental health assessment (formulation) is the vital starting point when planning subsequent care, and a bio-psychosocial approach must be employed including rigorous risk assessment and management. Discharge planning should involve CAMHS or the community team for people with learning disabilities (CTPLD) if appropriate.

 Learning activities

- Reflect upon the care that children with mental health problems have received in your clinical area and what skills are required to provide this care.
- What effect do you think a child who is self harming will have on the other patients on an inpatient paediatric ward, and what are the effects of being on the ward for the self-harming child?
- Reflect upon children with intellectual impairment who you have cared for. How were their health needs met in your clinical area? What consideration was given to their intellectual impairment in relation to aspects of their care such as pain assessment or preparation for procedures?

References and further reading

Ary DV, Duncan TE, Biglan A, Metzler CW, Noell JW, Smolkowski K (1999) Development of adolescent problem behaviour. *Journal of Abnormal Child Psychology* **27**: 141–150.

Burgess S, Hawton K, Loveday G (1998) Adolescents who take overdoses: outcome in terms of changes in psychopathology and the adolescents' attitudes to care and to their overdose. *Journal of Adolescence* **21**: 209–218.

Burke P, Cignof K (2000) *Learning Disabilities in Children*. Blackwell Science, Oxford: 34.

Department of Health (2001) *Valuing People: a new strategy for learning disabilities for the 21ˢᵗ century*. DH, London.

Essau C (2002) *Substance Abuse and Dependence in Adolescence*. Brunner-Routledge, Hove, Sussex.

Fox C, Hawton K (2004) *Deliberate Self-Harm in Adolescence*. Jessica Kingsley, London.

Gelder M, Mayou R, Cowen P (2001) *The Shorter Oxford Textbook of Psychiatry*. Oxford University Press, Oxford: 31–70.

Gillberg C (2003) *A Guide to Asperger's Syndrome.* Cambridge University Press, Cambridge: 17.

Hawton K, Kingsbury S, Steinhardt K, James A, Fagg J (1999) Repetition of deliberate self-harm by adolescents: the role of psychological factors. *Journal of Adolescence* **22**: 369–378.

Kelly P (2000) The dangerousness of youth-at-risk: the possibilities of surveillance and intervention in uncertain times. *Journal of Adolescence* **23**: 463–476.

Kerfoot M (1996) Suicide and deliberate self-harm in children and adolescents: a research update. *Children and Society* **10**: 236–241.

Kingsbury S, Hawton K, Steinhardt D, James A (1999) Do adolescents who take overdoses have specific psychological characteristics? A comparative study with psychiatric and community controls. *Journal of the American Academy of Child and Adolescent Psychiatry* **38**: 1125–1131.

Kroese B, Dewhurst D, Holmes G (2000) Diagnosis and drugs: help or hindrance when people with learning disabilities have psychological problems? *British Journal of Learning Disabilities* **29**: 26–33.

Lavery B, Siegel AW, Cousins JH, Rubovits DS (1993) Adolescent risk-taking: an analysis of problem behaviours in problem children. *Journal of Experimental Child Psychology* **55**: 277–294.

Lyon C, Pimor A (2004) *Physical Interventions and the Law.* British Institute of Learning Disabilities, Kidderminster, Worcestershire.

Simmonds J, McMahon T, Armstrong D (1991) Youth suicide attempters compared with a control group: psychological, affective and attitudinal variables. *Suicide and Life-Threatening Behaviour* **21**: 134–151.

Steinberg L (1996) *Adolescence*, 4th Edition. McGraw-Hill, New York.

World Health Organization (1992) *Tenth revision of the International Classification of Diseases and Related Health Problems (ICD-10).* WHO, Geneva.

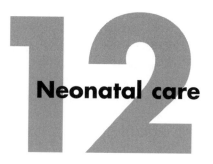

Neonatal care

Lynne Wainwright and Joyce Wood

Learning outcomes

- To develop an understanding of the common clinical reasons for neonatal high dependency care provision
- To develop an understanding of the respiratory, temperature, metabolic and nutritional assessment and management of neonates requiring high dependency care

Introduction

The aim of this chapter is to consider the management of neonates who require high dependency nursing care. The specific needs of neonates in relation to their immature physiology will be considered, especially concerning those who are born prematurely. The differences between problems seen in neonates at birth and those that present later will be discussed.

A neonate is defined as a newborn within the first 4 weeks of life. A baby born before 37 weeks' gestation is classed as premature. Currently the legal limit of viability is 24 weeks although some babies born at 23+ weeks are surviving.

The British Association of Perinatal Medicine (BAPM) (2001) noted high dependency care for neonates to include the following babies:

- Any baby of over 5 days of age or above 1000 g receiving NCPAP (nasal continuous positive airways pressure);
- Below 1000 g and not fulfilling any of the criteria for intensive care;
- Receiving parenteral nutrition;
- Having convulsions;
- Receiving oxygen and weighing below 1500 g;
- Requiring treatment for neonatal abstinence syndrome;
- Requiring specific procedures not fulfilling any criteria for intensive care – intra-arterial catheter or chest drain, partial exchange transfusion or tracheostomy care until supervised by parents;
- Requiring frequent stimulation for severe apnoeic episodes.

Neonates requiring high dependency care are therefore often either those who have spent time in intensive care or those who require admission to HDU shortly after birth. These infants will normally be nursed in a neonatal unit. However, in general if a baby has been home and requires admission to hospital they will be nursed on a children's ward. These babies are likely to have been born at term and to present with different problems. Many babies born prematurely will go on to require frequent hospital admissions after discharge from NICU.

Respiratory problems

Babies born at less than 30 weeks' gestation will often have inadequate levels of surfactant to allow them to breathe unaided. The level of support they require will depend on the gestation at which they were born and also whether the mother received antenatal steroids, which have been shown to mature the lungs (Lissauer and Fanaroff 2006). Surfactant is important in lowering surface tension in the lungs and prevents lung collapse at expiration, reducing the work of breathing.

The commonest cause of respiratory problems in neonates is respiratory distress syndrome (RDS). The majority of babies with RDS are those born prematurely, especially those born at less than 30 weeks' gestation. The most immature and sick babies will need to be intubated, given artificial surfactant and ventilated. Some may be adequately cared for on NCPAP with the aim being to provide support until the type 2 pneumocytes in the lungs produce enough surfactant. Many of these babies may develop chronic lung disease (CLD) defined by the need for oxygen at 36 weeks' gestation and a characteristic chest X-ray appearance (Rennie and Roberton 2002). They may go home under the care of the paediatric home care team, on low flow oxygen, which they may require for several months. They may require readmission to hospital with even a trivial upper respiratory tract infection causing respiratory distress.

Transient tachypnoea of the newborn can be seen in babies of any gestation, most commonly those born by elective caesarean section. It is caused by delayed clearance of lung fluid due to lack of hormonal response to labour and also the lack of being 'squeezed' through the vaginal canal, which helps to push out foetal lung fluid. These babies tend to present with tachypnoea, grunting and cyanosis. It is usually a mild condition that improves over the first 48 hours of life.

A further cause of respiratory distress in neonates of any gestation may be sepsis. Group B streptococcus is the most common bacterial infection in newborns. Respiratory syncytial virus can have devastating consequences for babies who were born prematurely or have lung or cardiac problems. These babies may present with non-specific symptoms such lethargy, apnoeas and bradycardias, desaturations, intolerance of feeds or unstable temperature (Rennnie and Roberton 2002). Respiratory support should be given as required and broad-spectrum antibiotics administered prior to results being obtained from blood cultures. Intravenous fluids may well be required and should be titrated to account for the possible hypoglycaemia that may present due to increased metabolic demands.

Care of the neonate requiring oxygen therapy or NCPAP

Oxygen can be administered to babies via headboxes, nasal prongs or via an incubator. Headboxes allow for accurate administration of oxygen and also of humidity but can provide a barrier between the baby and parents, and the inside can get very wet. Infants may also need to be removed for feeding and nappy changing, and nursing an active or distressed baby may be difficult.

Nasal prongs allow infants more freedom of movement and also mean that they can be fed more easily while receiving oxygen. It is, however, difficult to humidify the oxygen effectively and they can only be used for low flow oxygen up to 2 litres/minute.

Administration of oxygen via an incubator also allows for humidification. It can however be complicated to set up and to maintain the concentration. Larger term babies may also be very cramped in an incubator.

Nasal continuous positive airways pressure (NCPAP) is often used after extubation from ventilation or for babies whose condition is not severe enough to require intubation. It helps to maintain a function residual capacity in the lungs by delivering a constant pressure, thus reducing the work of breathing. Supplemental oxygen can be given if required. NCPAP is not always well tolerated by term infants and care needs to be taken due to the risk of pneumothorax if babies become distressed and fight the NCPAP.

NCPAP is most commonly delivered using a flow driver that utilizes fluidic flip technology deflecting the flow of gas during exhalation, so that the baby does not have to exhale against an incoming flow of gas. It can also be delivered using ventilators and an endotracheal or naso-pharyngeal tube, which can increase the work of breathing for a baby due to the difficulty of breathing through the narrow-bore endotracheal tube. When using via a flow driver NCPAP is administered to the baby using short nasal prongs or nose mask. In order to prevent excoriation of the nasal septum, nose care should be carried out at least 4-hourly, ensuring that there is no sign of skinbreak down. For babies who develop a sore nasal septum or for whom it is difficult to maintain an adequate seal with prongs, a nasal mask may provide relief. Prongs and masks are available in different sizes and it is important that the correct size is used. CPAP hats are also available in different sizes and these should be fitted carefully to ensure a good seal is achieved without causing too much pressure. As NCPAP has a tendency to force gas into the oesophagus as well as the trachea babies should always have an orogastric tube in situ to aid in decompression of the abdomen. The use of an orogastric rather than a nasogastric tube is preferable when babies are nursed on nasal prong oxygen or NCPAP to avoid blocking of the nostril. Babies may be fed while receiving NCPAP though care must be taken to avoid problems with tolerance of feeds. Babies on bolus feeds via a nasogastric tube should have the tube on high reflux between feeds to allow for the escape of excess gas. Some babies may more easily tolerate continuous nasogastric tube feeds using a syringe driver as this avoids overdistension of the abdomen. Small 'CPAP dummies' are available which allow babies to be comforted while on NCPAP.

All neonates requiring supplemental oxygen and/or NCPAP should have continuous monitoring of vital signs – heart rate, respiratory rate and oxygen saturation. The level of NCPAP being administered and the amount of oxygen required should also be recorded hourly. Capillary blood gas analysis should normally be taken at least once a day while a baby is on NCPAP; more frequently if the baby becomes unstable or displays signs of increased work of breathing, desaturation or bradycardia.

Babies are normally weaned off NCPAP when they are not having any episodes of bradycardia or desaturation and require a low level of supplemental oxygen. There is very little evidence regarding the best way to wean a baby from NCPAP. This is usually a gradual process, giving the baby a short time off initially, gradually increasing the time as the baby tolerates. Some babies initially appear to cope but become tired, require more oxygen and have bradycardias and desaturation. If a baby displays these symptoms they should be returned to NCPAP. It may also be appropriate to check a blood gas towards the end of the time off NCPAP to ascertain how well a baby is coping.

Hypothermia

Many neonatal problems will be much worse if the temperature is not maintained. Small babies, particularly premature and low birthweight babies, are unable to regulate their own temperature due to their immature hypothalamus and large surface area. Non-shivering thermogenesis is the main heat generation method in the first few weeks of life. This is achieved by metabolism of brown fat (found in the neck, between the scapulae and surrounding the kidneys and adrenals) which requires oxygen. Hypoxia therefore will adversely affect the neonate's ability to response to cold (Rennie and Roberton 2002). It is vital that care is taken to ensure that babies are nursed in a neutral thermic environment, maintaining their temperature as close to 37°C as possible. Heat can be lost by conduction, radiation, evaporation and radiation. Cold stress can have serious metabolic consequences for newborns and in the preterm infant these can be devastating (CESDI 2003). These consequences include – decreased surfactant production, hypoxia, increased anaerobic metabolism leading to acidosis, increased utilization of glucose leading to hypoglycaemia and, in the long term, poor growth. Cold babies can present with hypoglycaemia and/or grunting respirations, i.e. expiration against a partially closed glottis to try to maintain an adequate functional residual capacity. In addition to correction of the symptoms, correction of the temperature is vital and cold babies often require to be nursed in an incubator. Neonates may also present with unstable temperatures when septic, often becoming hypothermic as opposed to pyrexial.

Hypoglycaemia

Hypoglycaemia in the newborn is defined as a blood glucose level of less than 2.6 mmol/l (Merenstein and Gardner 2006). Most healthy term babies, despite the fact that they often feed infrequently in the first few days, are able to counter-regulate and will not suffer any ill effects (UNICEF 2008). Some babies are at high risk of hypoglycaemia. This includes babies with depleted glycogen stores, e.g. premature babies or intrauterine growth retarded babies, babies with serious infections, hypothermic infants or babies with metabolic disorders. In addition babies whose mothers have had poorly controlled diabeties during pregnancy may have high insulin levels leading to hypoglycaemia after delivery as the supply of glucose is reduced. Symptoms of hypoglycaemia include convulsions, lethargy, apnoea and hypotonia (Stephenson *et al.* 2000, Johnston *et al.* 2003). In high-risk babies feeds should be initiated as soon as possible, either orally or via nasogastric tube or, if gastric feeding is inappropriate, intravenous access should be obtained and an infusion of 10% dextrose commenced. A bolus of 3–5 ml/kg of 10% dextrose may be given if the initial blood glucose is low. Blood glucose should be checked after an hour to ensure that it has increased sufficiently. In a few babies 12.5% dextrose may be necessary to increase the blood glucose level sufficiently. Sick babies should have 6–12 hourly blood glucose measurements taken (Rennie and Roberton 2002). Babies requiring admission to HDU due to hypoglycaemia at times other than in the immediate postnatal period are likely to have feeding problems where their intake is inadequate – sometimes due to poor breastfeeding technique, or to be suffering from vomiting and/or diarrhoea or to have metabolic disease affecting glucose metabolism. In all cases it is important to increase the blood glucose level to above 2.6 mmol/l, and to maintain it between 3.6 and 6.5 mmol/l.

Case study 1: 2-week-old with hyperthermia and hypoglycaemia

Josh is a 2-week-old neonate born at 37+6 weeks' gestation weighing 2.7 kg and who went home 3 days ago bottle-feeding on demand. He has been admitted via the Emergency Department, sleepy and lethargic. Mum reports that he has not fed well for 24 hours and has had two moderate vomits.

On examination his temperature is 36°C, heart rate 110, respiratory rate 40, saturation 99% in air. His blood glucose is 2.1 mmol/ litre.

Management

Josh is cold and hypoglycaemic; though at present he is maintaining his oxygen saturation in air there is potential for this to become a problem due to cold stress. Josh should be placed in an incubator to increase his core temperature. Observations of temperature, heart rate, respiratory rate and oxygen saturation should be monitored continuously to enable quick assessment of his condition.

As Josh is hypoglycaemic a blous of 5 ml/kg of 10% dextrose should be given and an intravenous infusion of 10% dextrose commenced to maintain his blood sugar within normal limits.

A potential cause of Josh's problems is sepsis, and a blood culture and CRP should be taken. In the interim he may be commenced on prophylactic antibiotics which may be discontinued or changed according to sensitivities.

The possibility of a metabolic condition should be considered. This should all be explained to the parents, who should also be encouraged to care for Josh as they feel able. As his condition stabilizes he can be offered milk feeds and his intravenous fluids decreased as he tolerates milk and maintains his blood sugars. Feeds should be offered at intervals dependent upon how well he is able to tolerate them and on his blood sugar level.

Once his temperature has stabilized he can be moved into a cot and monitored to ensure he is able to maintain his temperature.

Jaundice

With the trend for babies to go home sooner after delivery, more babies are being readmitted to hospital requiring treatment for jaundice.

Jaundice is the yellow pigmentation of skin that occurs due to high plasma bilirubin levels. Bilirubin is the product from the breakdown of haem in the red blood cells. It is transported to the liver, bound to albumin as unconjugated bilirubin. In the liver it is conjugated, i.e. made water-soluble, to allow it to be excreted via the bile into the duodenum where some is reabsorbed and the rest excreted in the stools in the form of stercobilinogen. The kidneys excrete some of the reabsorbed conjugated bilirubin as urobilinogen. Only uncongugated bilirubin is toxic.

Physiological jaundice is very common in the neonatal period due to a large bilirubin production as a result of the shorter lifespan of neonatal red blood cells (40–70 days compared with 120 days in an adult), a high haemoglobin at birth (18–19 g/dl) and a low excretion of bilirubin, as the hepatic processes are immature with low levels of the liver enzymes necessary to conjugate bilirubin. In addition newborns have beta glucuronidase present in the gut from foetal life, which acts to deconjugate the conjugated bilirubin, allowing it to be reabsorbed into the enterohepatic circulation and excreted via the placenta and maternal liver. Around a third to a half of term babies will develop physiological jaundice (Johnston et al. 2003; Ebbesen 2004) with the number higher among preterm infants. In addition to immaturity of the conjugation process, the levels of serum bilirubin can be elevated due to other causes such as dehydration, sepsis or excessive red cell breakdown due to bruising from birth trauma. Physiological jaundice appears during the second day of life and reaches a peak by 3–7 days when the levels of bilirubin drop. Jaundice which manifests in the first 24 hours will be due to an underlying cause which was present in utero, for example rhesus or ABO incompatibility. Rhesus antibodies will often have been recognized during the antenatal period with some babies requiring in utero exchange transfusions. These babies will always be admitted to NICU for observation. Some babies also develop breast milk jaundice, the exact aetiology of which is unknown, though it may be due to high of levels of beta glucuronidase in breast milk.

This tends to have a later onset, peaking in the second or third week of life. It is generally thought to be harmless (Dent 2000) and breastfeeding should be continued.

Assessment and treatment of jaundice

Visual assessment of jaundice is often subjective and unreliable, however it is often the first reason a serum bilirubin level (SBR) may be requested in an otherwise well term baby. This is usually taken as a capillary blood sample via a heel prick.

In preterm babies SBRs may be checked more routinely due to the higher risk of jaundice that requires treatment. Levels of bilirubin requiring treatment are gestation and chronological age dependent. It is vital, therefore, that the correct chart is chosen when results are plotted.

Babies who are jaundiced may also be lethargic and disinterested in feeding. The treatment for babies whose SBR is above the 'treatment line' is phototherapy. Bilirubin absorbs light at the blue end of the spectrum (450 nanometres) and a number of processes cause it to change into a water-soluble state for excretion (Dent 2000). Babies requiring phototherapy should be nursed naked or wearing a 'bili nappy' and ideally be in an incubator in order to maintain their temperature. Eyes should be covered with a protective shield;, photochemical damage has been postulated. The phototherapy light should be placed 40–50 cm from the baby. Frequent repositioning of the baby may be required to ensure exposure of all areas of skin. No creams or lotions should be put on the skin. One of the side effects of phototherapy is the production of loose dark-green stools which are due to the increased excretion of unconjugated bilirubin via the gut (Stokowski 2006). Some studies have noted an increase in transepidermal water loss during phototherapy in addition to fluid loss from loose stools (Dent 2000; Stokowski 2006). This is most likely to be an issue in premature babies with fewer layers of epidermis. This may require extra fluids to be given to maintain the urine output and electrolyte balance. Assessment of serum bilirubin should be taken every 4–6 hours and plotted accurately on the bilirubin chart. Phototherapy should be switched off while blood is being taken. Once a baby has had two values below the treatment line, phototherapy can usually be stopped but the bilirubin should be monitored to ensure that it remains below the treatment line. It must be remembered that parents may find phototherapy distressing and they will need careful explanations and support.

It is not common for term babies to present with bilirubin levels that are above the exchange transfusion line. The aim of an exchange transfusion is to reduce the level of circulating bilirubin by removing blood from the infant's circulation in small amounts and transfusing the same amount of donor blood. Parental consent is required prior to the procedure. If possible the umbilical vessels should be used. However, this may not be possible in a baby who has been at home and presents via the Emergency Department or through the community midwife. In this situation the baby will require a peripheral arterial line and a peripheral venous line. The blood is removed in aliquots from the arterial line and replaced via the venous line. This may either be in aliquots or via continuous infusion calculated to go in at the same rate as the blood is removed. A full exchange transfusion may take 1–3 hours. During the exchange transfusion a baby should be continuously monitored and blood taken for blood gas, electrolytes (hyperkalaemia and hypocalcaemia may occur) and blood glucose. Accurate contemporaneous recording of blood in and out must be undertaken and an accurate fluid balance maintained to avoid fluid overload. Partial or dilutional exchanges may also be carried out on babies who present with neonatal polycythaemia, which Levene *et al.* (2000) define as a venous haematocrit over 65%, which equates to an Hb of 22 g/dl. Polycythaemia may cause problems due to a diminished blood flow through the small vessels.

Case study 2: 3-day-old infant with jaundice

Isabelle, a 3-day-old baby, was admitted via the community midwife with possible/suspected jaundice.

On admission she is pink with no obvious respiratory problems and her mother reports that she is breastfeeding quite well. Her respiratory rate is 50, heart rate 120, temperature 36.8°C and her weight is 3.2 kg.

A serum bilirubin (SBR) is taken which when plotted on the correct chart is just above the phototherapy line.

Management

As the SBR is above the treatment line Isabelle needs to receive phototherapy. This should be commenced as soon as possible to avoid the bilirubin level increasing further, risking development of kernicterus.

Isabelle should be nursed in an incubator to ensure that she can be nursed completely exposed to the lights, out of any draughts, and to maintain her temperature. Her eyes should be covered with phototherapy eye shields to avoid potential retinal damage and any creams must be removed from her skin. The phototherapy lights can then be switched on. This information should all be explained to parents to help alleviate their anxieties, as should the fact that Isabelle should still be encouraged to breastfeed. It should also be explained that in order to ensure that she gets the maximum effect of the phototherapy she should be placed straight back under the lights after a feed. Eye covers may be removed during feeds to facilitate bonding.

Observations should be recorded 4-hourly, with particular attention paid to temperature, as Isabelle may overheat due to being in the incubator and under the phototherapy lights. If this happens the incubator temperature should be adjusted. Fluid balance should also be monitored. If Isabelle is not feeding well, has loose stools, or if her urine output falls to below 1 ml/kg/hour she may require extra fluids, either intravenously or via a nasogastric tube. Her mother should be encouraged to express breast milk and the milk can then be given to Isabelle via the nasogastric tube; formula should only be used with the mother's consent. If this is not sufficient to maintain Isabelle's fluid balance or if she does not tolerate enteral feeds, intravenous fluids may be given. Four to six hourly SBRs should be taken and accurately plotted. Once two readings are below the treatment line phototherapy may be discontinued and a further SBR taken 6 hours later to ensure there is no rebound in level. During this time Isabelle can be dressed and nursed in a cot.

Blood sampling

Blood sampling is often necessary in babies who require high dependency care. As noted, these samples are necessary to determine blood gases, glucose levels and serum bilirubin levels as well as full blood count, urea and electrolytes and blood cultures. Some of these may be taken as venous or arterial samples but many will be taken as capillary samples via heel pricks (Figure 12.1). Care must be taken to ensure that the heel is only stabbed appropriately to avoid puncturing the calcaneous bone, which can cause osteomyelitis.

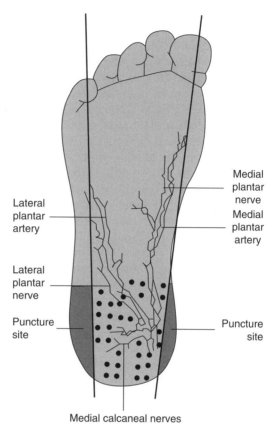

Lateral plantar artery

Lateral plantar nerve

Puncture site

Medial plantar nerve

Medial plantar artery

Puncture site

Medial calcaneal nerves

Figure 12.1 Anatomy of the foot, illustrating safe puncture sites.

Nutrition

Normal term babies are usually able to regulate their own intake when breast or bottle-feeding on demand. However, sick and preterm babies will be unable to do this.

Babies born before 34 weeks' gestation are unlikely to be able to coordinate sucking and swallowing adequately to be able to take their entire intake orally. These babies will require nasogastric tube feeding. The amount of enteral feed will be dependent on the gestational age and condition of the baby. Enteral feeds maybe gradually increased, reducing inravenous fluids as more enteral feed is given and tolerated. Feeds may initially be given continuously or hourly, increasing the time between as the baby progresses and tolerates milk. Nasogastric tubes should be aspirated 4–6 hourly both to check placement and to help determine how well feeds are being tolerated. Small aspirates should be returned via the nasogastric tube. However, large or bile-stained aspirates, vomiting or loose stools may indicate that the baby is not tolerating feeds, and feeds may need to be reduced or stopped. The baby's abdomen should also be observed for any signs of distension.

As a general rule a newborn's fluid requirements are:

- Day 1 – 60 ml/kg/day
- Day 2 – 90 ml/kg/day
- Day 3 – 120 ml/kg/day
- Day 4 onwards – 150 ml/kg/day

This will be altered dependent on the baby's blood results and clinical condition, e.g. urine output, blood sugar level and capillary refill time.

Neonates who need to be nil by mouth for short periods of time may be given intravenous fluids of 10% dextrose with additives of potassium and sodium according to the baby's electrolyte levels. However, babies requiring high dependency care may often have long periods when they need to be nil by mouth due to feed intolerance or the inability to feed due to illness or surgery. During these times total parenteral nutrition (TPN) is often given, ideally via a percutaneous long line or Broviac line in order to reduce the risk of extravasation injuries. This will ensure that the infant receives adequate calories during a period of rapid growth. TPN constituents will be prescribed according to the baby's U&E results. Infants receiving TPN should have blood glucose levels and urinalysis checked at least once a day. As enteral feeds are introduced and tolerated so the TPN rates can be reduced accordingly.

It is vital that mothers who are breastfeeding or who wish to breastfeed are encouraged to express their milk regularly and to freeze it for use once the baby is able to start feeding enterally. This will help to ensure that the breast milk supply is maintained. Breast milk is the best feed for all babies, especially those born premature or sick, with several studies having shown beneficial effects lasting into children from infant breastfeeding (King and Jones 2005). Babies who do not gain weight on expressed breast milk alone may require breast milk fortifier to be added to their feed once they are receiving full enteral feeds. In a few situations breastfeeding may not be recommended, e.g. for infants of mothers who are substance abusers or who are HIV positive. In these situations, or where mothers are unwilling to breastfeed, a suitable formula should be used. For premature babies this should be a specialist preterm formula. In some cases, for example babies who were born extremely preterm and who are at high risk of developing gut problems or who have had previous surgery, hydrolysed formula or donor breast milk maybe used (King 2005). For other babies the choice will be based on parental preference and also the condition of the baby since some babies may benefit from a specialist formula such as hydrolysed or high-energy milk.

Preterm babies who are not breastfed are often discharged on a specialized post-discharge formula containing the extra calories, vitamins and minerals necessary to promote growth. Breastfed babies will require vitamin and mineral supplements. Babies admitted due to respiratory infections may benefit from smaller volume feeds being given more frequently or to have at least some feeds given via nasogastric tube to allow them to rest.

Surgical problems

Most neonates who present with a surgical problem at birth will be cared for in a neonatal unit. However, some babies may require readmission either for problems that present later, e.g. pyloric stenosis, or who have problems following surgery. This may include adhesions or problems relating to poor feed tolerance. Introduction of feeds to babies who have had major gastrointestinal surgery should be undertaken gradually to monitor tolerance.

Babies who had gastrointestinal surgery for conditions such as necrotizing enterocolitis (NEC) or Hirschprung's disease in the immediate neonatal period requiring formation of a stoma may need to remain in hospital or require readmission at a later date to reverse the stoma. Necrotizing enterocolitis is most common in premature and intrauterine growth retarded babies. It is an inflammatory disease of the bowel. In some cases resting the gut and administering antibiotics may be enough, but in more serious cases surgery will be required to resect affected gut. An end-to-end anastomosis may then be possible but in some cases the gut is too badly affected and a stoma needs to be formed. The causes of NEC are multifactorial but the use of formula milk in very premature babies is felt to increase the risk.

Hirschprung's disease usually presents with failure to pass meconium, abdominal distension and vomiting. Where Hirschprung's disease is suspected a rectal biopsy is performed to determine the presence of ganglion cells in the bowel. The amount of bowel affected varies, with a few babies having involvement of the whole colon and small bowel. Rectal washouts may be used to decompress the intestine and remove meconium. Surgery may involve removal of aganglionic bowel and a primary pull through or formation of a temporary stoma in the ganglionic bowel, with later surgery to close it by pulling the ganglionic bowel through to the anus. Care of the peristomal skin is especially important in neonates due to the fragility of their skin. It is vital for the flange to fit as snugly around the stoma as possible with the minimum amount of skin showing. This is especially important if the baby has a high stoma in the small bowel as the losses will be particularly corrosive and skin breakdown will occur. All stoma output should be recorded and where there are large volumes of liquid losses these may need to be replaced intravenously. Involvement of the stoma nurse as soon as possible will help to ensure that the most appropriate care and appliances are used.

Babies who suffered severe NEC or long segment Hirschsprung's disease may be left with short gut syndrome, less than 40 cm of viable gut in a term infant (Levene *et al.* 2000). These babies have inadequate gut for normal absorption and may require long-term TPN, sometimes at home, usually via a surgically inserted central venous line. Infection and metabolic disturbances are common, as is cholestatic jaundice.

Pain

Assessment of pain in neonates is very important. All nurses caring for infants should have awareness of how to assess and manage their pain and of the consequences of untreated pain, for example physiological and neurological. Neonates exhibit chemical, behavioural and physiological responses to pain (East 2000). The nurse caring for the baby can see behavioural responses to pain which include facial expressions, crying and altered movements, and physiological responses which include changes in heart rate, respiratory rate, blood pressure and saturation. Chemical responses such in blood glucose cannot be seen and require analysis of blood samples. Non-pharmacological treatments for pain include swaddling and positioning; non-nutritive sucking using a dummy and sucrose can often be very helpful. In babies whose pain is not relieved by non-pharmacological measures, drugs may be used. These include paracetamol for mild to moderate pain through to morphine. As a major side effect of morphine is respiratory depression, it is not often used in babies who are not ventilated.

Conclusion

This chapter has discussed some of the problems with which neonates may present and the reasons why their care needs may differ from those of older children. Most sick newborns will be nursed in neonatal units, however those who have been at home prior to falling sick may be seen in emergency departments and admitted to high dependency areas in children's wards, therefore it is essential that nurses who work in such areas have sufficient knowledge of the physiology of newborns, their specific needs and the conditions with which they may present, to enable them to safely look after these babies.

Learning activities

- Review the principles of clinical assessment from Chapter 2 and discuss potential difficulties in applying these principles to neonates.
- Write a care plan for a 2-week-old with necrotizing enterocolitis in the neonatal high dependency unit.
- Formulate a discussion on the psycho-social impact of being a parent with a newborn child in the neonatal high dependency unit.

References and further reading

British Association of Perinatal Medicine (2001) *Standards for Hospitals Providing Neonatal Intensive and High Dependency Care*, 2nd Edition. www.bapm.org/publications/

CESDI (2003) 27/28 Project. The Stationery Office, London.

Dent J (2000) Haematological problems. In Boxwell G (ed.) *Neonatal Intensive Care Nursing*. Routledge, Oxford.

East P (2000) Pain and comfort in neonatal intensive care. In Boxwell G (ed.) *Neonatal Intensive Care Nursing*. Routledge, Oxford.

Ebbesen F (2004) Jaundice in the newborn infant. www.bloodgas.org (accessed 10 July 2008).

Johnston P, Flood K, Spinks K (2003) *The Newborn Child*, 9th Edition. Churchill Livingstone, London.

King C and Jones E (2005) The benefits of human milk for the preterm baby. In Jones E, King C (eds) *Feeding and Nutrition in the Preterm Infant*. Churchill Livingstone, London.

King C (2005) Enteral feeding. In Jones E, King C (eds) *Feeding and Nutrition in the Preterm Infant*. Churchill Livingstone, London.

Levene M, Tudehope D, Thearle J (2000) *Essentials of Neonatal Medicine*, 3rd Edition. Wiley Blackwell, London.

Lissauer T, Fanaroff A (2006) *Neonatology at a Glance*. Blackwell, London.

Merenstein G, Gardner S (eds) (2006) *Handbook of Neonatal Intensive Care*, 6th Edition. Mosby, St Louis, MO.

Rennie J, Roberton N (2002) *A Manual of Neonatal Intensive Care*. Arnold, London.

Stephenson T (2000) *Pocket Neonatology*. Churchill Livingstone, London.

Stokowski L (2006) Fundamentals of phototherapy for neonatal jaundice. *Advances in Neonatal Care* 6(6): 303–312.

UNICEF (2008) *Guidance on the Development of Policies and Guidelines for the Management of Hypoglycaemia of the Newborn*. www.babyfriendly.org.uk (accessed 10 July 2008).

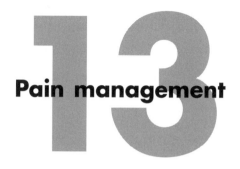

Pain management

Andrea Cockett

Learning outcomes

- To develop an understanding of the importance of an appropriate pain assessment process
- To develop an understanding of different methods of pain management both pharmacological and non-pharmacological
- To develop an understanding of sedation techniques that may be useful in the high dependency setting

Introduction

Pain management is an important part of the care that is provided for a child requiring high dependency care. The child may be in pain due to their illness and they may also have to undergo painful procedures while in the high dependency unit. Inadequate pain management can lead to children feeling helpless, anxious, irritable and depressed and their coping skills may be undermined (Weisman *et al.* 1998). Children become sensitized to pain through changes in the nervous system, and once pain has been undertreated, it becomes harder to treat, even with the same noxious stimulus. Children who experience extreme procedural pain can develop post-traumatic stress disorder (Weisman *et al.* 1998).

The physiology of pain

Having an understanding about the physiological processes that are occurring during a painful episode enables nurses to treat the pain in the most appropriate manner. Multimodal pain management is the gold standard in paediatric services. Acute pain is the physiological response of the body to danger. Nociception is the term used to describe the normal processing of pain and the body's response to it (McCaffery and Pasero 1999).

Nociception has four main components:

- transduction
- transmission
- perception
- modulation.

Transduction of pain is the result of nociceptor stimulation. The nociceptors (nerve endings) of Aδ and C fibres within the nervous system respond to noxious stimuli. These stimuli are categorized into three main types:

- mechanical (pressure, swelling, tumours, incisions);
- thermal (burns);
- chemical (neurotransmitters, toxic substances, ischaemia, infection).

Nociceptors are present in both internal and external organs. They can be found in the skin, muscles, bones and also in the liver and gastrointestinal tract. The Aδ and C fibres are responsible for the transduction of pain within the nervous system. The fibres have different properties and are responsible for different types of pain transduction. Aδ fibres are large, myelinated fast transmission fibres which transmit well-localized, sharp pain sensations.

C fibres are smaller, unmyelinated, slower fibres which transmit diffuse burning and aching sensations. The noxious stimulus can be internal or external. The stimulus causes the release of chemical mediators from the cells involved. These chemical mediators include substance P, bradykinins, histamine, potassium, prostaglandins and serotonin. These chemical mediators activate and/or sensitize the nociceptors to the noxious stimuli. In order for a pain impulse to be generated, an exchange of sodium and potassium ions (depolarization and repolarization) occurs at the cell membranes. This results in an action potential and generation of a pain impulse.

Transmission of pain occurs in three stages. The Aδ and C fibres transmit the signal to the spinal cord. It then travels up the spinal cord to the brain. It is then transmitted via the brain stem to the thalamus and higher levels within the brain.

Perception of pain occurs within different areas of the brain; there is no one area of the brain responsible for pain perception. The reticular system is responsible for our motor and autonomic response to pain. The somatosensory cortex identifies the location and intensity of the pain and the limbic system is responsible for our emotional and behavioural response to the pain.

Modulation of pain involves the changing or inhibiting of the pain in the spinal cord. The pathways involved in the modulation of pain are called the descending modulatory pain pathways. These are responsible for our individual response to pain. The pathways release neurotransmitters in response to pain. These neurotransmitters include encephalins and endorphins alongside serotonin and noradrenaline. Individuals will release varying amounts of neurotransmitter, which explains the difference in individuals' responses.

Pain assessment

Pain assessment is an integral part of any clinical assessment undertaken of a sick child. Kuttner (1996) describes trying to assess someone else's pain as like trying to speak a foreign language that you don't understand. Untreated or undertreated pain can have a detrimental effect on a child's clinical condition (Cummings *et al.* 1996). The literature suggests that some children, particularly those who are having difficulty communicating due to their age or cognitive ability, are at risk of being left in pain (Twycross 1998). The aims of pain assessment are to define the severity of the child's pain, select appropriate analgesia to treat the pain and then evaluate the effectiveness of that analgesia. It is important that the correct approach is used when assessing pain and that an objective approach is always utilized. In order for pain assessment to be successful it is important that the following underlying philosophies are in place:

- Children are listened to and believed.
- Children and their families are viewed as partners in care.
- Care is individualized and holistic.
- Care is family centred.
- A collaborative, multi-professional approach is provided by knowledgeable professionals.
- Attention is paid to the organizational issues and systems that enable effective pain management to take place (Royal College of Nursing 1999a).

Pain assessment should be undertaken as soon as is reasonable within the process of the clinical assessment. Pain should also be assessed if there is a change in clinical condition such as tachycardia or hypotension or if the child starts to complain of intense pain. The assessment needs to be undertaken at regular intervals, usually when other clinical parameters are being measured, so as not to unduly disturb the child. Assessment should also always be completed after the administration of analgesia, to measure its effectiveness.

Pain assessment should be individualized for each child so if possible a pain history should be obtained on admission. This should cover whether the child has had any experience of pain before, what that experience was like, any treatments that were utilized and also the language that the child and family use to describe pain (Royal College of Nursing 1999a). Any cultural factors that may affect the pain experience should also be documented.

Indicators of pain

Evidence is clear that the most reliable source of pain assessment in children is the child's self report (Almond 1999). If self report is not possible then behavioural signs are considered to be the next most accurate method for assessing children's pain (Almond 1999). Physiological signs can be utilized as part of a holistic pain assessment but they are not accurate alone and can be misleading as other factors may be affecting them (Stark 1998).

Many factors influence the pain experience that children will have. These include:

- age
- gender
- understanding
- learning
- family's response to pain
- previous pain experiences
- social reinforcement
- control issues
- culture
- beliefs, attitudes and expectations
- psychological state (Twycross 1998).

Neonates and infants may display the following behavioural responses to pain:

- crying
- change in facial expression
- motor responses

- change in posture
- change in activity level
- undue quietness
- restlessness
- change in appearance such as skin colour.

No measure should be used in isolation for this age group and gestational age must be taken into account when undertaking the assessment.

Young children may be able to self report their pain. Four is considered to be the age at which self report of pain becomes accurate and reliable (Almond 1999). Behavioural responses in this age group include:

- crying
- change in facial expression
- motor responses
- change in body posture
- change in level of activity
- change in appearance.

Older children on the whole should be able to self report. If this is not possible due to their clinical condition then behavioural measures similar to those used for younger children can be utilized successfully.

Pain assessment tools

Pain should always be assessed using a validated pain assessment tool that is suitable for the age of the child. There are a number of tools that are suitable for children who are unable to self report due to their clinical condition, or self-report tools that can be utilized by those children able to undertake an assessment.

Neonatal and infant pain scale
This tool was developed at the Children's Hospital of Eastern Ontario (Lawrence and Alcock 1993) and is recommended for infants of less than 1 year. A score of 3 or more indicates pain (Table 13.1). Utilizing the tool effectively means being able to interpret the behaviours demonstrated by the infant.

FLACC (face, legs, activity, cry, consolability)
This tool is suitable for use in children aged 2 months to 7 years so it is very versatile (Merkel et al. 1997) (Table 13.2). The minimum score is 0 and the maximum score is 10.

Wong-Baker faces pain rating scale
This scale (Figure 13.1; Wong et al. 2001) is a self-report scale that is suitable for use in children aged 3 and above. It can also be used for

Table 13.1 Infant and neonatal pain scale. Source: Lawrence and Alcock (1993) The development of a tool to assess neonatal pain. *Neonatal Network, Journal of Neonatal Nursing* **12**: 59–66. Used with permission. Copyright Elsevier.

Pain assessment		Score
Facial expression		
0 – Relaxed muscles	Restful face, neutral expression	
1 – Grimace	Tight facial muscles; furrowed brow, chin, jaw, (negative facial expression – nose, mouth and brow)	
Cry		
0 – No cry	Quiet, not crying	
1 – Whimper	Mild moaning, intermittent	
2 – Vigorous cry	Loud scream; rising, shrill, continuous (Note: Silent cry may be scored if baby is intubated as evidenced by obvious mouth and facial movement)	
Breathing patterns		
0 – Relaxed	Usual pattern for this infant	
1 – Change in breathing	Indrawing, irregular, faster than usual; gagging; breath holding	
Arms		
0 – Relaxed/Restrained	No muscular rigidity; occasional random movements of arms	
1 – Flexed/Extended	Tense, straight legs; rigid and/or rapid extension, flexion	
Legs		
0 – Relaxed/Restrained	No muscular rigidity; occasional random leg movement	
1 – Flexed/Extended	Tense, straight legs; rigid and/or rapid extension, flexion	
State of arousal		
0 – Sleeping/Awake	Quiet, peaceful sleeping or alert random leg movement	
1 – Fussy	Alert, restless and thrashing	

younger children if the practitioner feels they are cognitively able to understand the tool.

Original instructions: Explain to the person that each face is for a person who feels happy because he has no pain (hurt) or sad because he has some or a lot of pain. *Face 0* is very happy because he doesn't hurt at all. *Face 1* hurts just a little bit. *Face 2* hurts a little more. *Face 3* hurts even more. *Face 4* hurts a whole lot. *Face 5* hurts as much as you can imagine, although you don't have to be crying to feel this bad. Ask the child to choose the face that best describes how he is feeling.

Table 13.2 The FLACC: a behavioral scale for scoring postoperative pain in young children. Source: Merkel *et al.* (1997) *Pediatric Nursing* **23**(3): 293–297. Used with permission. Copyright The Regents of the University of Michigan.

Category	Scoring		
	0	**1**	**2**
Face	No particular expression or smile	Occasional grimace or frown, withdrawn, disinterested.	Frequent to constant quivering chin, clenched jaw.
Legs	Normal position or relaxed.	Uneasy, restless, tense.	Kicking, or legs drawn up.
Activity	Lying quietly, normal position moves easily.	Squirming, shifting back and forth, tense.	Arched, rigid or jerking.
Cry	No cry, (awake or asleep)	Moans or whimpers; occasional complaint	Crying steadily, screams or sobs, frequent complaints.
Consolability	Content, relaxed.	Reassured by occasional touching hugging or being talked to, distractible.	Difficulty to console or comfort

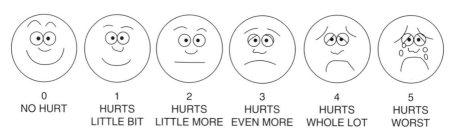

0	1	2	3	4	5
NO HURT	HURTS LITTLE BIT	HURTS LITTLE MORE	HURTS EVEN MORE	HURTS WHOLE LOT	HURTS WORST

Figure 13.1 Wong-Baker faces in pain rating scale. Source: Wong DL, Hockenberry-Eaton M, Wilson D, Winkelstein ML, Schwartz P (2001) *Essentials of Pediatric Nursing*, 6th Edition. Used with permission. Copyright Mosby.

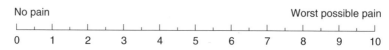

No pain   Worst possible pain

0   1   2   3   4   5   6   7   8   9   10

Figure 13.2 Visual analogue scale.

Brief word instructions: Point to each face using the words to describe the pain intensity. Ask the child to choose face that best describes own pain and record the appropriate number.

Visual analogue scale
A visual analogue scale (VAS) uses a linear representation of pain and is used for self report in older children (Figure 13.2). The line is always 10 cm long and starts at 0 with no pain and finishes at 10 with the worst possible pain.

A VAS can only be used for children who are numerate, so this excludes most children under the age of 5. Visual analogue scales tend to be used for older children or adolescents (Twycross 1998).

Managing procedural pain in children

Children requiring high dependency care often require multiple painful procedures during assessment and treatment of their condition. It is important that procedural pain is assessed and managed well to aid the child's recovery (Cummings *et al.* 1996).

The aims of procedural pain management are to:

- prevent and minimize the pain as much as possible;
- ascertain what the child's expectations are and correct them if necessary.

Anticipatory anxiety plays a large part in the experience of procedural pain for children and it is very important to deal with this effectively prior to the procedure starting (Von Baeyer *et al.* 2004). There is a direct correlation between anxiety and the intensity of the pain experienced. An integrated approach has been found to be the best way of managing procedural pain (Liossi 2002). This requires the practitioner to use both pharmacological and non-pharmacological methods to achieve a manageable procedure for the child. Using an integrated approach has the following benefits for the child and family (Kazak *et al.* 1998):

- It decreases anxiety prior to procedures.
- It provides a sense of mastery over stressful situations.
- It encourages the active involvement of parents.
- It provides significant pain control for procedures.
- It promotes effective coping for subsequent procedures.

When choosing what techniques are suitable the practitioner needs to take into consideration the following characteristics of the child and the situation (Kazak *et al.* 1998):

- age;
- previous experience with this or other procedures;
- expected intensity and duration of pain;
- anxiety levels of the child and parents, and their ability to cope;
- physical state.

Special situations to be taken into account:

- neonates;
- children with communication or behaviour problems;
- children with physical disability;
- children who are undergoing or likely to undergo repeated procedures.

Parental involvement in managing procedural pain

Anxiety of adults present at a procedure can affect the child's anxiety and coping levels so it is important that parents are prepared appropriately but also that they participate in the procedure appropriately. Parental activity can be divided into two categories, useful and not so helpful (Blount *et al.* 2003).

Useful parental activity:

- Non-procedural talk (e.g. birthday parties, pets, favourite activities, etc.);
- Distraction methods (e.g. favourite music, toys, games, bubbles, clowns, etc.);
- Breathing techniques;
- The adult prompting the child to use coping strategies.

Not-so-useful parental activity:

- Making reassuring comments (e.g. 'It'll be all right');
- Making empathic comments (e.g. 'I know it's hard');
- Apologizing (e.g. 'I'm sorry you have to go through this');
- Criticizing (e.g. 'You're being a baby');
- Bargaining with the child (e.g. 'I'll get you a playstation if you let them do it');
- Providing explanations during the procedure;
- Giving the child control over when to start the procedure (e.g. 'Tell me when you're ready);
- Catastrophizing and becoming agitated (Blount *et al.* 2003).

Non-pharmacological techniques

> **Tip**
>
> Preparation of the child and other adults present at the procedure is paramount.

Preparation of the child should involve an explanation that is age and clinical condition appropriate. This should include information about the procedure itself and the sensations that may be experienced by the child during the procedure. There should be an opportunity for the child to ask questions if their clinical condition allows this. If possible the child should be allowed some choices in the way in which the procedure is conducted. This will allow the child to feel some control over the situation. These choices can include whether to lie down or sit during a procedure but should not involve complete control over the procedure. The clinical condition of the child and the urgency of the procedure must be taken into consideration at all times (Kolk *et al.* 2000).

Techniques that can be used during the procedure involve the following (for older children):

- distraction
- story-telling
- guided imagery.

Distraction

Distraction is an essential component of any procedural pain management. The distraction needs to be relevant to the age and cognitive level of the child. Distraction techniques are also useful for involving parents and allowing the child to feel that they have some control over the situation. Ideally the distraction technique should be practised for 5 to 10 minutes before the procedure. The underlying principle of distraction is that we all have a limited amount of mental capacity to allocate to various tasks, at any given time, and distracting means the child concentrates on that rather than the pain. Distraction techniques are most helpful when a child's pain is mild to moderate (difficult to concentrate when pain is severe).

Distraction is helpful because:

- Child does not require training;
- Works with infants and older children;
- Involvement of parents;
- Minimal training for staff.

Types of distraction that can be used:

- Treasure box – have a box with small stickers in that can be given to the child during or after the procedure.
- Blowing bubbles – relaxes children by slowing and deepening the breath.
- Counting – have the school-age child count during a difficult part of the treatment.

- Singing – a child who has not gone too far in fear or anxiety may be soothed with singing or being sung to.
- Diversional talk – talking about the weather, your last holiday, the child's family, etc. in a comforting, rhythmic voice can be calming.
- Soothing touch – rhythmic touch alleviates loneliness and fear and promotes relaxation.
- Pop-up books – reading and using the pop-ups can allow mind stimulation and distraction.
- Hide-inside books – using the 'Where's Wally' theme, for example, may distract the child and alleviate some anticipatory pain.

Story-telling
Story-telling is a useful distraction technique for procedural pain. It is useful on two levels for distracting the child and also for providing parents with a role during the procedure. It can be used in conjunction with play and with other distraction techniques.

Guided imagery
Guided imagery is a useful technique that can be used effectively even with quite young children. It is a cognitive intervention that uses the imagination and children are particularly good subjects for it as they respond naturally and spontaneously (Langley 1999). Children are asked to imagine a favourite place and then guided through the place by asking them to use all their senses. It is important for the effectiveness of the imagery that they are asked to describe the warmth of the place, the colours that they see and the sounds that they hear. This enables the child to hold a detailed image in their mind, so providing the best level of distraction from the procedure. The child controls the image by choosing he place they want to describe but the skill of the practitioner is in leading the child through the image and asking them to describe it in detail.

Sucrose and non-nutritive sucking
Sucrose and non-nutritive sucking can be used for procedural pain management in neonates and infants. This is the administration of a sucrose solution to the infant, with or without the use of a dummy, to promote sucking behaviours. The physiological basis for this is that sucrose and pain relief are interrelated through the body's endogenous opioid system that provides natural analgesia. Endogenous opioid mediation occurs following activation of receptors at the tip of the tongue (Gibbins *et al.* 2002).

The pain-relieving effect is not found in infants given sucrose via a nasogastric tube but only in those who receive it orally. If used in conjunction with a dummy then it is effective in reducing both the intensity and response to pain (Stevens *et al.* 2004). The opioid response appears to be mediated by taste only and the effect of sucrose can be reversed by naloxone, an opioid antagonist. This suggests that it has a similar effect to opioid analgesics. It is thought that the analgesic effect comes from inhibition of the pain transmission at spinal level. There may also be the release of endorphins from the hypothalamus. Systemic absorption is not required for the sucrose to be effective. The optimum time for administration is 2 minutes before the painful procedure and the effect of the sucrose lasts for up to 5 minutes, with the peak effect being achieved at 2 minutes (Mitchell and Waltman 2003).

Tip

Non-nutritive sucking is the provision of a dummy to promote sucking behaviours.

The pain-relieving effect of this appears to be from the stimulation of orotactile and mechanoreceptors. It is most effective when combined with sucrose but can be used alone (Gibbins *et al.* 2002).

Pharmacological methods

There is a wide range of pharmacological methods that can be used to alleviate procedural pain. When deciding which method to choose it is important to consider the following factors:

- Age and clinical condition of the child;
- The length of the procedure;
- The expected level of pain intensity.

A combination of pharmacological methods can be used such as a local anaesthetic and a systemic analgesic.

Topical anaesthetic creams

Topical anaesthetic creams such as EMLA and Ametop are very useful for managing procedural pain. EMLA contains lignocaine and takes about an hour to work. Ametop contains amethocaine and takes 30 to 45 minutes to work. Some studies have shown Ametop to be more effective than EMLA (Arrowsmith and Campbell 2000; Boyd and Jacobs 2001) for venepuncture in children. Their most common use is in venepuncture, cannulation and lumbar puncture. Side effects are rare but sometimes a skin reaction can occur.

Local anaesthetic agents

Anaesthetic agents can also be injected into sites for procedural pain management or sprayed onto sites. Common drugs used include lignocaine and bupivacaine. In order to minimize pain the smallest needle possible should be used for their administration and a topical agent should be applied first. There is a small risk of systemic uptake of the drug so attention should be paid when administering the drug to ensure that there is no inadvertent vascular administration. Side effects of local anaesthetic agents include lightheadedness and dizziness. There can also be a local reaction if the child is allergic to the agent.

Nitrous oxide

Nitrous oxide is most commonly used as Entonox®. This is a self-administered inhaled mixture of 50% nitrous oxide and 50% oxygen. It provides effective short-term analgesia with minimal risk of adverse effects (Bruce and Franck 2000). It is commonly used in childbirth but has been shown to be effective in children for use during reduction of fractures and laceration repair. Entonox® has analgesic, sedative and anxiolytic effects. Because the drug is inhaled it has a very rapid onset and also a very rapid cessation of action. This makes it ideal for procedural pain management. In order for nitrous oxide to be used effectively the child must have the cognitive ability to understand how to use the inhalation mechanism. It is most effective when it is used in conjunction with a systemic analgesic agent and a psychological intervention (Bruce and Franck 2000). Parental consent is required and appropriate resuscitation equipment must be available. The child should be observed at all times to check their level of consciousness.

Safe delivery of nitrous oxide:

- Preferably the child should not have eaten for 1 hour before administration.
- Administer 100% oxygen for 2 to 3 minutes before and after the procedure.
- Maintain verbal contact with the child at all times.
- Monitor heart rate, respiratory rate, pulse oximetry and consciousness level.
- Provide 100% oxygen if the child suffers an adverse effect.
- Ensure the full effect of the nitrous oxide is felt by the child before starting the painful procedure.

The most common side effects of nitrous oxide are nausea and dizziness. More serious side effects include oversedation and airway obstruction.

Nitrous oxide should not be used in children where the following conditions are diagnosed or suspected:

- pneumothorax
- head injury
- suspected drug or alcohol misuse
- diabetic coma or metabolic illness
- air embolism
- decompression sickness.

Morphine

Morphine is the drug of choice for severe procedural pain. Care must be taken when it is administered to ensure that the child is closely observed for side effects, particularly respiratory depression. For this reason it is preferable if children are monitored with pulse oximetry if morphine is administered.

Sedation

Sedation can be necessary during procedures if a combination of non-pharmacological and pharmacological techniques are not enough for the procedure to be carried out safely and with minimal distress to the child.

The following drugs are the most widely used for managing procedural sedation in children.

Midazolam

Midazolam is a short-acting sedative and anxiolytic. It has no analgesic properties so must always be used in conjunction with an appropriate analgesic agent. It can be administered by a number of different routes including intranasally which makes it a versatile drug. The reversal agent is flumazenil and this must always be available if midazolam is being administered.

Side effects of midazolam include respiratory depression, a heightened reaction (agitation) and nasal irritation if given via this route. Doses for different routes are listed in Table 13.3.

Ketamine

Ketamine is an analgesic and deep sedative agent. Its use is limited to procedures where deep sedation is necessary because of the age of the child or the type of procedure. It should only be used when a paediatric anaesthetist is present and full airway support and resuscitation facilities are close to hand. It cannot be used on infants younger than 6 months and must be used with caution in children with upper respiratory tract infections as it can cause laryngospasm.

Table 13.3 Midazolam doses and routes of administration.

Route	Dose	Maximum dose
Intravenous	0.05–0.15 mg/kg	5 mg (titrated slowly to this maximum dose)
Oral	0.5 mg/kg	15 mg
Rectal	0.25–0.5 mg/kg	10 mg
Intranasal	0.2–0.5 mg/kg	10 mg

Holding children

Managing procedural pain can be difficult in certain situations and it may become inevitable that a child will need to be held for a procedure. Holding children for procedures should always be a last resort and all other avenues should have been considered prior to holding taking place (Lambrenos and McArthur 2003). The Royal College of Nursing (1999b: 4) defines holding as 'immobilization which may be by splinting or by using force. It is a method of helping people, especially children, with their permission, to manage a painful procedure quickly and effectively'.

Important factors to consider when deciding to hold a child for a procedure include:

- Have you explained the procedure adequately to the child and family?
- Do you have consent of the child and family to hold the child?
- Is the procedure urgent and therefore cannot be postponed?
- Is there an appropriately trained member of staff present to hold the child?
- Does the parent wish to hold the child or be shown a safe holding technique by a member of staff?

It is very important that the consent of the child and family are sought before holding and that this is documented. It is also important that staff are trained in safe holding techniques and the procedure to be followed if a decision is made to hold a child. Debriefing the child and family following the procedure should always happen.

Continuing pain management

In addition to managing procedural pain it is important that ongoing acute and chronic pain are also managed for children requiring high dependency care. A comprehensive pain management programme needs to be in place that combines assessment, management and evaluation of both pain and pain management strategies for each child. Evidence shows that children with medical as well as surgical conditions can suffer from acute pain (Royal College of Nursing 1999a).

Pharmacological management of continuing pain

There are several analgesics that can be used to manage acute pain and also different modes of delivery.

Paracetamol

Paracetamol is an analgesic used to treat mild to moderate pain. It acts by inhibiting prostaglandin synthetase centrally. It is most commonly administered orally or rectally. A loading dose should be given when it is being used for pain relief. The loading dose is:

- 20 mg/kg orally; 30 mg/kg rectally.

The oral maintenance dose can vary but usually a 15 mg/kg dose is used.

The total amount given by whichever route in 24 hours must not exceed 90 mg/kg/day (60 mg/kg/day in a baby) (BMJ Publications 2008). Paracetamol should be used with caution in renal and hepatic failure. The dosage interval should be increased in renal failure and large doses should be avoided in hepatic failure. An overdose of paracetamol can result in liver damage and liver failure.

Non-steroidal anti-inflammatory drugs

Non-steroidal anti-inflammatory drugs (NSAIDs) have analgesic, anti-inflammatory and antipyretic properties. They act by inhibiting the enzyme cyclo-oxygenase (COX) and the synthesis of prostaglandins. There are two COX enzymes and inhibition of COX-2 will have mainly analgesic and anti-inflammatory effects. COX-1 is thought to be responsible for most of the adverse effects. Ibuprofen and diclofenac are the NSAIDs most often used in acute and postoperative pain in children. Ibuprofen can be used as an alternative to paracetamol and is less likely than the other NSAIDs to cause gastrointestinal side effects. NSAIDs can be used in combination with paracetamol.

Adverse effects of non-steroidal anti-inflammatories
The main adverse effects of NSAIDs are:

- gastrointestinal discomfort, nausea, and diarrhoea;
- occasionally bleeding and ulceration;
- headaches, dizziness, vertigo, confusion;
- fluid retention;

- hypersensitivity reactions such as bronchospasm, rashes;
- local burning, itching or occasional bleeding that may occur with NSAID suppositories.

Opioid drugs

Opioid drugs are extremely useful in the treatment of severe pain in children.

Oral opioids include codeine phosphate and morphine. Opioids should be given intravenously for severe pain either using nurse-controlled analgesia (NCA) or patient-controlled analgesia (PCA). The most commonly used opioid administered in this way is morphine. Opioids produce their effect by acting at opioid receptors which are found in the brain, spinal cord and sites in the central nervous system, including urinary and gastrointestinal tracts, lung and peripheral nerve endings. There are three principal types of opioid receptors: mu (OP3), delta (OP1) and kappa (OP2). Opioids in common use act primarily at the mu receptor sites.

Adverse effects of opioids

- Respiratory depression
- Excessive sedation
- Nausea and vomiting
- Pruritis
- Constipation
- Urinary retention
- Muscle spasms.

Opioids should be used with caution in children with respiratory depression and head injury. Care should be taken with head injury patients as opioids can change the papillary responses that are a vital part of the neurological assessment.

The two most commonly used opioid drugs are codeine phosphate and morphine.

Codeine phosphate is normally administered orally. Morphine can be administered in a number of different ways. The most common methods of administration for continuing pain are orally or by continuous intravenous infusion. If an intravenous infusion is going to be utilized then it is important to ensure that the child is pain free at the start, so a bolus dose may need to be given.

Patient-controlled analgesia

Patient-controlled analgesia (PCA) is a patient-triggered, computer-controlled, parenteral morphine infusion pump which allows the child control over the analgesia. It has been used successfully in children as young as five but this requires individual assessment. Any child can have PCA, provided they are able to understand the concept and able to press the button. It is very important that the mechanism of the PCA is explained to both the child and family prior to the child using the pump. It is also very important that the child is pain free during this explanation and when initially being connected to the pump. If the child is not pain free at this point the use of PCA is unlikely to be successful as the child's pain will not be brought to a manageable level. The PCA pump can be used in a number of ways:

- Continuous background infusion with top-up bolus doses available;
- Only on demand bolus doses.

With any protocol there will be a lock-out period whereby a child cannot receive another bolus dose for a period of time. This is to prevent accidental overdose. It is important that records are kept of how often the child is demanding a bolus dose and how often they are receiving the dose. This is to monitor the effectiveness of the infusion. Other observations that need to be recorded include:

- pain score
- sedation score
- respiratory rate
- heart rate
- saturation levels.

It is very important that only the child controls the infusion, so parents need to be aware that the child must press the button for the bolus dose.

Nurse-controlled analgesia

Nurse-controlled analgesia (NCA) is indicated for children who cannot understand or operate the PCA. NCA allows a bolus dose to be given by the nurse prior to short procedures or when the continuous infusion is insufficient. The former is a quicker way to control pain than increasing the infusion rate.

The observations required by the child are the same as those for PCA.

Epidural analgesia

Epidural analgesia can be used very successfully with children. It is of particular use for children who are undergoing thoracic, spinal or lower limb procedures. In most units children with epidural infusions in progress are nursed in high dependency units. This is due to the complications that can arise from the use of epidural analgesia.

The spinal nerves consist of an anterior and posterior root. The anterior root contains the motor nerves which travel out of the spinal cord. The posterior root carries sensory fibres into the spinal cord (Dickenson 1995). These sensory fibres transmit touch, temperature and pain signals into the spinal cord. The nerve roots begin and end in the in the anterior and posterior horns of the spinal cord. They cross over the subarachnoid space where they are bathed in cerebrospinal fluid (CSF) and then they travel across the dura mater and the epidural space to form the main spinal nerve trunks (Dickenson 1995).

The epidural space contains fat, blood vessels and nerves. The epidural catheter is placed between the dura mater and the vertebral arch. This means that it does not come into direct contact with the CSF.

Two drugs are commonly used in epidural analgesia: opioids and local anaesthetics. The opioids administered via the epidural catheter diffuse across into the CSF and bind to the opiate receptors in the dorsal horn of the spinal cord. Some opioid is also absorbed systemically via the epidural veins. The local anaesthetic component of the epidural analgesia works primarily on the nerves in the epidural space. Selective blockage of muscle, sensory and sympathetic impulses can be achieved depending upon the concentration of the anaesthetic and the duration of its use (Chrubasik and Chrubasik 1995). Catheters are usually placed at the lumbar or caudal level in infants and young children as this is technically easier. Thoracic placement is reserved for older children. The most commonly used drugs are:

- opioid: morphine or fentanyl;
- local anaesthetic: bupivacaine or ropivacaine.

Complications of epidural analgesia can be divided into three different components.

Catheter-related complications

- Migration
- Occlusion
- Shearing
- Epidural haematoma
- Neural injury/paraesthesia
- Postdural puncture headache

Opioid-related complications

- Respiratory depression
- Hypotension

- Nausea and vomiting
- Urinary retention
- Pruritus
- Nightmares
- Myclonic movement

Anaesthetic-related complications

- Hypotension
- Sensory block
- Motor block
- Pressure ulcers
- Altered level of consciousness
- Seizures
- Dysrhythmia.

Due to the complications of epidural analgesia, close observation of the child is paramount. The following observations need to be recorded:

- heart rate
- blood pressure
- respiratory rate
- temperature
- pain assessment
- neurological assessment
- pulse oximetry.
- Inspection of the catheter site looking for:
  - leakage
  - drainage
  - haematoma
  - pain
  - erythema.

An epidural protocol should be available in every clinical area where children are cared for. This should include information about standard dosages, training required and the procedure to be followed for changing infusions.

Conclusion

This chapter has discussed the care of children requiring high dependency and their pain. Strategies for managing procedural pain have been described and also the needs of children with ongoing pain. The importance of accurate and timely pain assessment has been discussed and the various analgesia options available have been detailed.

Learning activities

- Reflect on a patient whose pain you have assessed and treated with analgesia. Review the information in this chapter and decide if you would do anything differently in a similar situation in the future.
- Reflect on a situation where you have needed to sedate a child. Think about the effectiveness of this sedation.

References and further reading

Almond C (1999) Acute paediatric pain – assessment and management. *Emergency Nursing Journal* **2**(3): 22–24.

Arrowsmith J, Campbell C (2000) A comparison of local anaesthetics for venepuncture. *Archives of Disease in Childhood* **82**: 309–310.

Blount RL, Seri LG, Benoit MA, Simons LE (2003) Effective coping: essential but ignored in pediatric pain assessment. *Suffering Child* October (4).

BMJ Publications (2008) *BNF for Children.* http://bnfc.org/bnfc/

Boyd R, Jacobs M (2001) EMLA or amethocaine (tetracaine) for topical analgesia in children. *Emergency Medicine Journal* **18**(3): 209–210.

Bruce L, Franck L (2000) Self administered nitrous oxide (Entonox®) for the management of procedural pain. *Paediatric Nursing* **12**(7): 15–19.

Chrubasik S, Chrubasik J (1995) The use of patient-controlled epidural analgesia for acute and chronic pain. *Pain Reviews* **2**: 29–37.

Cummings EA, Reid GJ, Finley GA, McGrath PJ, Ritchie JA (1996) Prevalence and source of pain in paediatric patients. *Pain* **68**: 25–31.

Dickenson AH (1995) Spinal cord pharmacology of pain. *British Journal of Anaesthesia* **75**: 193–200.

Gibbins S, Stevens B, Hodnett E, Pinelli J, Ohlsson A, Darlington G (2002) Efficacy and safety of sucrose for procedural pain relief in preterm and term neonates. *Nursing Research* **51**(6): 375–382.

Hockenberry MJ, Wilson D (2009) *Wong's Essentials of Pediatric Nursing*, 8th Edition. Mosby, St. Louis, MO.

Kazak AE, Penati B, Brophy P, Himelstein B (1998) Pharmacologic and psychologic interventions for procedural pain. *Pediatrics* **102**(1 Pt 1): 59–66.

Kolk AM, van Hoof R, Fiedeldij Dop MJ (2000) Preparing children for venepuncture: the effect of an integrated intervention on distress before and during venepuncture. *Child: Care, Health & Development* **26**(3): 251–260.

Kuttner L (1996) *A Child in Pain: what to do, how to help.* Hartley & Marks, Vancouver BC.

Lambrenos L, McArthur L (2003) Introducing a clinical holding policy. *Paediatric Nursing* **15**(4): 30–33.

Langley P (1999) Guided imagery: a review of effectiveness in the care of children. *Paediatric Nursing* **11**(3): 18–21.

Lawrence J, Alcock D (1993) The development of a tool to assess neonatal pain. *Neonatal Network, Journal of Neonatal Nursing* **12**: 59–66.

Liossi C (2002) *Procedure-Related Cancer Pain in Children*. Radcliffe Medical Press, Oxford.

McCaffery M, Pasero C (1999) *Pain: a clinical manual*. Mosby, St Louis, MO.

Merkel SI, Voepel Lewis T, Shayevitz JR, Malviyas A (1997) The FLACC: A behavioural scale for scoring pain in young children. *Pediatric Nursing* **23**(3): 293–297.

Mitchell A, Waltman P (2003) Oral sucrose and pain relief for preterm infants. *Pain Management Nursing* **4**(2): 62–69.

Royal College of Nursing (1999a) *The Recognition and Assessment of Acute Pain in Children*. RCN, London.

Royal College of Nursing (1999b) *Restraining, Holding Still and Containing Children*. RCN, London.

Stark K (1998) Paediatric pain management. *Australian Nursing Journal* **6**(4): Suppl. 1–4.

Stevens B, Yamada J, Ohlsson A (2004) Sucrose for analgesia in newborn infants undergoing painful procedures. *Cochrane Database of Systematic Reviews* Issue 3.

Twycross A, Moriarty A, Betts T (1998) *Paediatric Pain Management: A multidisciplinary approach*. Radcliffe Medical Press, Oxford.

Von Baeyer CL, Marche TA, Rocha EM, Salmon K (2004) Children's memory for pain: overview and implications for practice. *Journal of Pain* **5**(5): 241–249.

Weisman SJ, Bernstein B, Schechter NL (1998) Consequences of inadequate analgesia during painful procedures in children. *Archives of Pediatrics & Adolescent Medicine* **152**(2): 147–149.

Wong DL, Hockenberry-Eaton M, Wilson D, Winkelstein ML, Schwartz P (2001) *Essentials of Pediatric Nursing*, 6th Edition. Mosby, St Louis, MO.

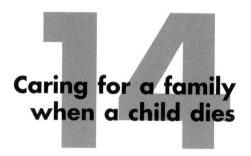

Caring for a family when a child dies

Andrea Cockett

Learning outcomes

- To develop an understanding of the issues surrounding bereavement
- To develop an understanding of the nursing care required by the child and family when a child dies
- To develop an understanding of the legal issues surrounding a child's death

Introduction

Caring for a child and family when a child dies can be one of the most difficult roles that a nurse will undertake. When working in high dependency care it is more likely that this situation will be encountered than when working in a normal ward environment. The nature of the patient's condition also means that death may be sudden and unexpected following an acute illness or traumatic injury. Caring for a dying child and their family is both a privilege and a challenge (Cook 2000).

Bereavement

In order to care for a family in this situation it is useful to have an understanding of current bereavement theory. Traditional bereavement theory postulates that grief has stages that the bereaved will go through. Parkes (1986) describes four stages of bereavement. These are: an initial response of numbness shock and disbelief; a second phase of grief, searching for meaning, anger, guilt, sadness and fear; a third phase of despair; and then a final phase of adjustment, acceptance and gaining a new identity. The difficulty with this type of model is that it views grief as a problem that must be overcome rather than as a normal life process. A more recent theory of bereavement is the dual process model (Stroebe and Schut 1999). This model (Figure 14.1) promotes the idea that the bereaved person must cope with the experience of the loss itself and the changes that result from the loss.

In this model the bereaved are described as being in either loss-orientated mode or restoration-orientated mode. The bereaved person can move between these modes at different times and they are not 'set'. The loss-orientation phase is the part that encompasses the grief work. This involves looking at photographs of the deceased, crying and longing for the deceased. The restoration-orientated mode is about acknowledging the secondary changes that a bereavement imposes and the 'work' that needs to be undertaken to create a new life from the previous one. This involves learning new tasks and making new friendships. Using a bereavement model such as this one enables the nurse to see that the bereaved person is not in a fixed path and that there is dynamism between the different tasks that a bereaved person needs to undertake.

Other factors that need to be taken into consideration when caring for a bereaved family are cultural issues and gender. Culture has been shown to play a part in how bereaved individuals behave (Walter 1999) so consideration must be given to cultural practices that may seem alien

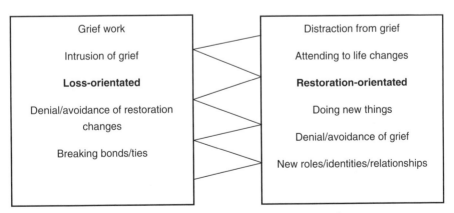

Figure 14.1 Loss-oriented and restoration-oriented roles in the grief process.

to the individual nurse. Gender also plays a role in coping with loss. Male and female responses are different but not isolated to either gender, so males can have a 'female' response and vice versa. The female response to grief is 'intuitive' and involves the expressing and sharing of emotions while the male response is 'instrumental' and involves trying to figure out what to do (Doka and Martin 1998).

Providing care to a bereaved family

Certain guiding principles need to be followed when caring for a family during a bereavement. The first and foremost of these is that the family needs to be treated in an individualistic way. It is vital that the care they receive takes account of their cultural, spiritual and religious needs. It is also of key importance that care is coordinated across the multidisciplinary team and across services. The family will need ongoing care and support once they have left the acute hospital setting and communication between primary, secondary and tertiary services needs to be excellent.

One of the aspects of care that needs to be considered in a high dependency unit is the witnessing by parents of resuscitation. The Resuscitation Council (UK) (1996) recommends that relatives are allowed to be present at resuscitation. They suggest that the relatives should be supported by an appropriately trained member of the healthcare team. The evidence surrounded witnessed resuscitation suggests that relatives benefit in a number of ways (Robinson et al 1998):

- They feel that everything is being done for the patient.
- They feel that their presence may influence a positive outcome.
- In follow-up, relatives who witnessed resuscitation had fewer symptoms of grief and distress.

In order to facilitate the presence of parents at a resuscitation procedure the following issues need to be addressed within the high dependency unit:

- Staff must receive educational input on the effect of having parents present both on themselves and the parents.
- An experienced member of staff must be allocated to look after the parents at all times.
- All actions, equipment and decisions must be explained to the parents.
- It should be made clear to them that they can leave at any time.
- The parents must be allowed the opportunity to be debriefed afterwards whatever the outcome (Royal College of Nursing 2002).

Sudden and unexpected death is extremely traumatic for families. Admission to hospital and transfer to a high dependency area can give parents the impression that their child will be cured. When death is unexpected there has been no preparation or gradual acceptance that the child's death is inevitable, as there may be during a chronic illness. Parents in this situation are often in denial about what has happened and can experience severe feelings of guilt. They can spend a lot of time trying to understand the events that led to the child's admission to hospital and the events that have happened since admission. These feelings can be particularly severe if the child has died following an accident or a very short illness. Parents have very little time in which to adapt to the reality of what has happened and communication is key during these situations. It is also very important that contact with the child is maintained during an unexpected and sudden death. This will help the parents to deal with the reality and to help them feel empowered to have some control over what happens to their child.

Communication is crucial when a child has died. Studies of parents' experiences of breaking bad news have identified factors that they considered to be important (Krahn *et al.* 1993; Field *et al.* 2003):

- Not being told alone, ensuring that a partner or family member is with them.
- Being able to touch their child during the interview with the medical staff.
- The healthcare professionals touching the child with obvious care and respect.
- The healthcare professionals recognizing that the parents are primarily responsible for the child.
- Showing caring compassion and a sense of connection with the family.
- Healthcare professionals being willing to show their own emotions.

In order to meet the needs of families at this distressing time it is important that all of the healthcare professionals involved observe similar standards when communicating with families. Time for the parents to ask questions both immediately after the event and subsequently at a follow-up appointment should be available. Parents should not feel in any way rushed in their discussions with staff. A private secure area should be provided for parents to stay in and also to meet with staff. A parent should not be given bad news when alone unless it cannot be avoided. Staff should wait for the partner or another family member or friend to arrive before discussing issues with the parents. Written material concerning the procedures that will be followed and the information given should be available to the parents. This is very important as parents will not remember much of the information given to them verbally, and in the case of a post-mortem being required or a coroner being involved they will need detailed information. Other factors to consider are whether it would be better to have an interpreter present if English is not the parents' first language and the need for clear understandable language to be used.

If a child's death is imminent or they have just died after a failed resuscitation attempt then the staff need to ask the parents if they would like a member of their religion to be called. All Trusts will have religious staff available at all times of the day and night. If the child is an infant and the parents are Christian then they may wish to have the child baptized. If a priest or chaplain cannot get to the hospital in time it is possible for a member of staff to carry out an emergency baptism. Baptism is not usually carried out after death.

Practical care required by the child

When a child has died there are certain practical procedures sur-rounding the care of the child's body that need to be carried out. It is very important that parents feel in control of what happens after their child has died. Initially parents should be allowed to spend as much time as they would like with their child, either with a member of staff present or alone. The only time that parents cannot be left alone with their child is if non-accidental injury is suspected. In this case a member of staff must remain with the child at all times. It is also important that the needs of other family members are taken into consideration at this time, particularly siblings. Parents should be asked what they would like to do about other relatives seeing and being with the child.

Parents should also be consulted about the amount of involvement they would like in providing the practical care that their child needs after death. If they wish to be involved in this aspect of their child's care then they need to be supported by an experienced member of staff. All monitoring equipment should be turned off and all medical devices should be removed. If there is to be a postmortem or the case is referred to the coroner then medical devices should be left in situ. They should be disconnected from any infusions or drainage bags and spigotted as close to the skin as possible. All dressings should be replaced and covered with a waterproof dressing to stop leakage. The chid will need to be washed after death and should be dressed in their own clothes. Their own toiletries should be used to wash them. If the child normally wears a nappy then a clean nappy should be put on. Their bladder should be expressed to ensure no urine is present.

The child should be laid flat with their head in a central position to stop any marking of the face. The child must have an identity band on. Keepsakes should be offered to the parents including photographs of the child, a lock of hair and palm and footprints. These can only be taken with the consent of the parents. If they feel unable to make a decision at the time the staff can offer to take the keepsakes and keep them in the child's notes for a later date. Parents should be able to accompany their child to the mortuary and many parents wish to carry their child, particularly if they are young.

It is possible for parents to take the child home with them if there is not going to be a postmortem and the case is not referred to the coroner. If the parents wish to take the child home they can either take the child themselves or an undertaker can collect the child and take them to their home. If the parents are going to take the child then they will need to have the death certificate and also a letter explaining the situation in case they are involved in a traffic accident during the journey home. It is advisable that neither parent should drive and that a friend or relative does this for them.

Once a child has died and left the unit the staff are responsible for ensuring that all appropriate personnel are informed including the health visitor and the GP.

The staff should ascertain how parents are going to travel home if they are not taking their child with them. They should also ensure that the parents have all the relevant information that they need. This should include:

- Information about what will happen to their child now;
- That they may return to see their child whenever they want and how to arrange this;
- Written information about registering the death and how to arrange a funeral;
- Any keepsakes.

Legal issues

Parents will need to be given the child's death certificate before they leave the hospital. It is good practice for parents not to be expected to return for a death certificate. Normally deaths are registered in the area in which the child has died. It can be done in the home area of the family but this can delay the paperwork so leading to a delay in funeral arrangements. If there is to be a postmortem or the case is referred to the coroner then the parents will not be able to have the death certificate immediately. Deaths must be registered within 5 days. Many registrars' offices will make special arrangements for parents to ensure that they are not left waiting around to register a death Often if staff telephone the registrar's office in advance the parents will be seen straight away.

Postmortems

Postmortems can be requested by the medical staff, the coroner or the family. Written consent is always required unless the postmortem is requested by the coroner. Cases are referred to the coroner for the following reasons:

- After an accident or injury;
- During a surgical operation;
- Before recovery from an anaesthetic;
- If the cause of death is unknown;
- If the death is sudden or unexpected (sudden infant death);
- If the death was violent or unnatural (suicide, drug overdose).

Once a death is referred to the coroner they will decide if a postmortem is required and if any further investigation is warranted. If the coroner decides a postmortem is required then only the coroner can issue the death certificate.

When consent for postmortem is requested from families by the medical staff then it is very important that parents fully understand what will happen. In particular they need to know that tissue or organs may be kept for further examination.

Organ donation

Some children may be suitable to become organ donors. If this is the case then they will normally be transferred to a paediatric intensive care unit where their care will be managed by the organ donor team. Children who have died from their illness can still donate tissue such as heart valves and eyes. Organ donation has been shown to be of great comfort to families of children who have died (Rodrique et al. 2008) so should be considered for all suitable children even if they cannot donate whole organs.

Ongoing care

Ongoing care is very important for bereaved families. If a postmortem has been carried out then the parents should be offered an appointment to see the consultant as soon as the results are available. All parents should be offered a follow-up appointment with their child's consultant following a death. The child's health visitor and GP should arrange to see the parents and referral to a bereavement counsellor should be arranged. It is also important not to forget the care required by siblings when a child has died. Siblings will respond differently to the death of a brother or sister depending on their age. The death should be explained to them in language that they understand and ideally they should be given the opportunity to see their dead sibling. Follow-up of the family should take account of the needs of siblings and separate counselling may need to be arranged for them. It is very important that the health visitor or GP follows up and visits the family shortly after the bereavement to ensure that the needs of siblings have not been forgotten.

Conclusion

This chapter has discussed some key issues involved in caring for a child who has died. It is important that staff are familiar with their own Trust's policies and procedures in relation to death and bereavement. Care provided for families at this very difficult time can leave a lasting impression that can be significant in the family's grieving journey.

References and further reading

Cook M (2000) The dying child. In Williams C, Asquith J (eds) *Paediatric Intensive Care Nursing*. Churchill Livingstone, London.

Doka KJ, Martin T (1998) Masculine responses to loss: clinical implications. *Journal of Family Studies* **4**(2): 143–158.

Field MJ, Behrman RE (eds) (2003) *When Children Die: improving palliative and end-of-life care for children and their families*. National Academies Press, Washington, DC.

Krahn GL, Hallum A, Kime C (1993) Are there good ways to give 'bad news'? *Pediatrics* **91**(3): 578–582.

Parkes CM (1986) *Bereavement Studies of Grief in Adult Life*. Tavistock, London.

Resuscitation Council UK (1996) *Should Relatives Witness Resuscitation?* Resuscitation Council, London.

Robinson SM, Mackenzie-Ross S, Campbell-Hewson GL, Egelston CV, Prevost AT (1998) Psychological effect of witnessed resuscitation on bereaved relatives. *Lancet* **352**(9128): 614–617.

Rodrique JR, Cornell DL, Howard RJ (2008) Pediatric organ donation: what factors most influence parents' donation decisions. *Pediatric Critical Care Medicine* **9**(2): 180–185.

Royal College of Nursing (2002) *Witnessing Resuscitation: guidance for nursing staff*. RCN, London.

Stroebe M, Schut H (1999) The dual process model of coping with bereavement: rationale and description. *Death Studies* **23**: 197–224.

Walter T (1999) *On Bereavement: the culture of grief*. Open University Press, Buckingham.

Index